PARKINSON'S DISEASE GUIDE
FOR THE NEWLY DIAGNOSED

PARKINSON'S DISEASE

Guide for the Newly Diagnosed

Understanding the Disease,
Managing Your Symptoms
& Navigating Treatment

PETER LeWITT, MD

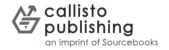

callisto
publishing
an imprint of Sourcebooks

Copyright © 2020 by Callisto Publishing LLC

Cover and internal design © 2020 by Callisto Publishing LLC

Interior and Cover Designer: Erik Jacobsen

Art Producer: Tom Hood

Editor: Lia Ottaviano

Production Editor: Rachel Taenzler

Callisto and the colophon are registered trademarks of Callisto Publishing LLC.

Published by Callisto Publishing LLC C/O Sourcebooks LLC

P.O. Box 4410, Naperville, Illinois 60567-4410

(630) 961-3900

callistopublishing.com

Printed and bound in China

OGP 2

CONTENTS

INTRODUCTION

You or your loved one has just received a diagnosis of Parkinson's disease. What's next? You probably have a lot of questions and may be feeling confused, angry, frustrated, or sad—there's no right way to feel when you receive a serious medical diagnosis like Parkinson's disease (PD). It's normal to feel overwhelmed during this time, but my hope is that this book will give you the tools to help you feel more in control and better prepared to navigate this disease.

The diagnosis of PD often brings a flood of fears and uncertainties that can be devastating for one's sense of self and well-being. Sometimes the diagnosis is the final chapter in months or years of relatively minor warning signs and symptoms. These signs can include shakiness, slurred speech, handwriting that trails off, or walking with a different gait that makes it difficult to keep up with others. The inkling that something is wrong can also be quite subtle and intermittent, such as a slight tremor or clumsiness; sometimes the signs are so unnoticeable to oneself that it takes the observations of others for one to notice them. However, it is the physician's diagnosis of PD that brings an entirely new set of challenges. It can seem like a judge's reading of a prison sentence, especially with the gravity implied by the word *disease*. For those living with PD, their perception of the disorder can vary; some have the luxury of viewing their symptoms as a small nuisance, and others view the disorder as much more, perhaps as a future disability. However, well-informed PD patients will come to realize that this diagnosis is neither the prelude to "imprisonment" nor a path toward accelerated mortality. They will realize, instead, that the diagnosis of PD means the arrival at a new world of health and lifestyle changes that, fortunately for most people, is more on the side of a nuisance than a life-altering disability.

In any case, your acquaintance with the diagnosis and reality of PD was probably unwelcome. In my case, I was introduced to PD in a very different context that arose just when I completed my three-year residency training in adult neurology. At the time, I was searching for a specific direction in my new professional career that would combine gaining further expertise in current therapeutics with the emerging opportunities of research developments pointing to new treatments—including the hope for a cure for PD and other neurological conditions. For three years after completing neurology training, I pursued this additional experience as a research fellow at the National Institute of Neurological Disorders and Stroke (NINDS), the branch of the massive National Institutes of Health enterprise that includes PD research. After that training and research experience in Bethesda, Maryland, I moved to Michigan, where during more than 30 years of clinical and research practice at various institutions, my career goals haven't changed. I'm still committed to making the most of the current treatment options, exploring new therapeutic opportunities through clinical trials and laboratory research, and developing a better understanding of this malady so that people may be able to live better lives with PD in the future. With the constant march forward of new developments in medical technologies and treatment options, many, if not most, people today are able to achieve better management of their symptoms so that they can lead full and productive lives despite the intrusion of PD. You'll find many of the tools, techniques, and strategies to cope with PD in this book, and, I hope, you'll be able to integrate them into your own life.

One of my goals in working with people who have PD, especially those who are newly diagnosed, is to emphasize that they are entitled to *realistic optimism*. Let me repeat that, because it is important to keep this concept in mind as your mantra: Those who live with PD are entitled to realistic optimism. By this statement, I mean that most people can overcome the impositions of PD, including impaired mobility, tremors, and even the stigma of a change in outward appearance. Not everyone with PD will be so fortunate, and the quality of life from person to person can be difficult to predict, but, given what we know about this disorder, the majority will benefit from today's effective therapies. Of course, it's difficult to make generalizations about every aspect of PD, because it comes in several different forms, with symptoms varying from patient to patient, and each person's experience and personal "grit" in coping with PD can vary greatly. Especially on that first day when the diagnosis is pronounced, the path ahead never seems to be a straight course. It probably looks a little different for each patient. But no matter the circumstances surrounding your diagnosis, the severity of your symptoms, or the treatment options available to you, it's important to maintain a full measure of realistic optimism. Much of the quality of life in living with PD depends on an attitude toward overcoming the diagnosis. Some persons may respond with fear, anger, and sadness and undergo a shutdown. Alternatively, another path is to focus on self-education to learn how to maintain a healthy, productive life and take charge of the diagnosis.

Every physician getting to know a PD patient should recognize that the diagnosis is a shock, often bringing with it an overwhelming sense of dread. Carefully listening to and acknowledging the details of PD can be very challenging at such a time. What some physicians communicate to their patients might be jumbled jargon and a less-than-calming vision of PD. That leads to one of the purposes of this book: to serve as a guide for how to improve the quality of patient–physician conversations and to provide guidance on how to ask the right questions. Beyond the information that I will share with you in these pages, there are several other important steps a patient can take to take charge of PD and thrive with it. One of the best ways to gain confidence in living with this disorder is to equip yourself with knowledge through further reading and Internet searching. However, it's important to keep in mind that not all content out there on the web is positive or healthy; too much, especially on disreputable sites that may provide incorrect information, can lead to needless anxiety and overthinking. Products sold as if they offer a cure should be viewed with strong suspicion, of course. You can find many informative, authoritative websites in the Resources section at the end of this book (see page 108).

The shock of reckoning with the diagnosis of PD calls for a jump-start with critical information and a reminder that you are not alone. Many others (as you will read later, about 1 percent of persons over the age of 60) are on the same journey. The chapters ahead will discuss the nature of PD, its symptoms, and treatment options and provide guidance on how to navigate daily life with family, friends, and work colleagues. We'll also delve into how to make sense of your diagnosis, the medical professionals who will help guide you each step of the way, and how to integrate lifestyle choices that can make it easier to live with this condition. As you'll learn in this book, staying healthy with PD involves more than just keeping up with your medications; well-planned meals, structured exercise plans, paying attention to your quality of sleep, and working to ensure good communication with others (especially your care team, which we'll discuss later) are important in mastering PD. Another crucial component of taking charge of PD is networking with others affected with PD. You'd be surprised how much comfort and support you can find in strangers who share your or a loved one's diagnosis; look for local support groups or groups on social media. In fact, PD was one of the first medical conditions to foster the support group movement that now seems universal for nearly every medical diagnosis. There is an informative and inspiring event held every three years by the aptly named World Parkinson Congress. During this meeting, attended by thousands of patients and their families from just about everywhere, the sense of a global PD community is uniquely fostered. Here in the United States, dozens of national and regional groups also support the PD cause, such as the American Parkinson Disease Association, the Michael J. Fox Foundation for Parkinson's Research, and the Parkinson's Foundation.

My goal for this book is to acquaint you with key details of PD as it stands today in order to prepare you to live with PD and also to introduce you to its possible future, when better symptomatic treatments and the possibility of a cure are likely. In the chapters ahead, we'll learn more about the disorder itself, the symptoms associated with it, effective medications and treatments, and guidance and tips on how to live your best life with PD.

CHAPTER 1
The Facts about Parkinson's

In this chapter, we'll cover pertinent information about the stages, types, and possible causes of PD. If you or your loved one has been newly diagnosed with PD, this is a great place to start for better understanding this diagnosis and what it means. Much research into the manifestations of PD has been done, but we still have a lot to learn about its origins and causes. Even the diagnosis of PD may require a second opinion in many cases, since its symptoms can overlap with those of other neurological disorders. With all that has been learned about PD over the past two centuries, there is also plenty of misinformation about the disorder, so it's important to seek out up-to-date and authoritative sources for valid information (such as those you will find at the end of this book in the Resources section starting on page 108).

What Is Parkinson's Disease?

In England in 1817, a very observant general practitioner strolling the streets of London noticed some subtle, strange behaviors exhibited by a few of the people he passed by. In these individuals, he observed movements that were slower than normal, tremors (the shaking of limbs), and other distinctive physical impairments that he characterized in great detail. He wrote a short book on this topic, which he described as the "shaking palsy." Later in the 19th century, other physicians reading his monograph and recognizing his insight in the discovery of this affliction attached to it the name of the author, James Parkinson, MD. Two centuries after its publication, *An Essay on the Shaking Palsy* (1817) is still a source of useful information. Although the medical terminology has evolved, the observations of James Parkinson serve as a reminder that what we encounter today is essentially the same condition. Dr. Parkinson described persons in words that bring to life the PD experience. Reading this essay today provides observations that accurately convey many of the core features of what we now know as PD. For example, Dr. Parkinson noted that, in patients afflicted with the "shaking palsy," handwriting can be smaller than usual and trails off, "fail[ing] to answer with exactness to the dictates of the will." Dr. Parkinson also detailed other telltale signs of PD: buttoning a shirt can require a great deal of effort, and walking often lacks a fluid arm swing and even spacing of steps. Rhythmic to-and-fro movements (tremors) may cause an otherwise resting hand to shake involuntarily. As Dr. Parkinson observed, and as we know today, the total picture of motor impairments among people with PD can vary greatly. Sometimes they remain exclusively one-sided, affecting only the right or left limbs, and lacking in tremor, though for others, a tremor with the limbs at rest is the major symptom. Variability in symptoms is one of the corner-stone characteristics of PD, which can add to the challenge of PD diagnosis, since symptoms can fluctuate from day to day and even from hour to hour.

When PD patients think back to the very first clue they noticed that indicated something wasn't right, many times it wasn't out-wardly apparent or obvious. Sometimes it is an internal sense of tremor that's invisible to others, or a curious, unfamiliar sensation such as unexplained tingling or warmth in an arm. The earliest features of PD can often be too subtle for even an experienced clinician to make a confident diagnosis. Awareness about PD has greatly increased in the past two decades. Even now, many cases are misdiagnosed as other conditions, simply because physicians lack full knowledge about the disorder. Sometimes patients with very mild symptoms are referred to an orthopedist because their decreased arm swing during walking led to an impression of a "frozen shoulder." Diagnosing PD sometimes can be difficult, as many of its warning signs and symptoms closely mimic those of other neurological disorders. Shaking hands are sometimes dismissed as anxiety or familial-type ("essential") tremors, and both problems can be found in a PD patient. Preceding the onset of PD's motor symptoms, some-times by years, can be problems with an unexplained decline in olfaction (sense of smell) and an increase in active dreaming, in which the patient may talk or move during the dream stage of sleep. Based on the many forms PD can take and the widely varying symptoms through which it can present itself, it seems clear that the diagnosis of PD presents some challenges, especially in its earliest manifestations. A skilled diagnostician

Parkinson's Disease Statistics

How many PD patients are there in the United States? Although we don't have a precise figure, there are likely several million people living with the disorder, since an estimated 1 percent of people over the age of 60 are affected. About 5 percent of people living with PD are younger than 50 years of age. Even though a diagnosis of PD initially may feel like a prison sentence, it is by no means a death sentence. PD does not reduce life span, so the average patient lives with this disorder for 15 or more years. Men are more likely than women to receive a PD diagnosis, at a 3:2 ratio. PD is probably underdiagnosed, even in people who receive regular medical care, in large part because its signs and symptoms are often attributed to "old age" or can be ignored altogether, especially if the symptoms are mild or intermittent. About 5 to 10 percent of PD cases, especially those diagnosed with early-onset PD (younger than age 60), are thought to have a genetic basis for their Parkinsonism. Parkinsonism is the umbrella term given to the clinical syndrome that is found in PD but also in several related disorders.

and sometimes a second opinion by another clinician may be necessary for establishing whether PD is present or not. If this all seems overwhelming, it can be. An understanding of the full spectrum of PD is constantly evolving as physicians continue to learn more about the disorder and they, just like their patients, aim for realistic optimism with each diagnosis.

So what is the modern understanding of this disorder? PD is classified as a neurodegenerative disease. This means that PD involves the progressive loss of neurons within discrete regions of the brain. The neurons, or nerve cells, lost in PD have specific functions linked to their signaling chemicals, particularly one called dopamine. Dopamine is a member of a class of chemicals (called neurotransmitters) that signal between nerve cells. Specifically, neurotransmitters direct the electrical functions of cells to generate output patterns that control movement. In PD, because of a loss of the functional units (nerve cells and dopamine), the electrical brain circuitry that controls movement can be changed so that proper function is impaired.

In the case of PD, the changes developing in nerve cells preceding their loss are characterized by the arrival of abnormal structures called Lewy bodies. Lewy bodies can't be seen in scans of a living person's brain but are readily evident in brain tissue examined under a microscope outside of the body. Neuroscientists view these types of changes as uniquely human, since they do not arise spontaneously elsewhere in the animal kingdom. Chemical analysis of Lewy bodies reveals that they are mostly comprised of large aggregates of an otherwise normal protein called alpha-synuclein. Alpha-synuclein is normally present within healthy nerve cells, but in PD it specifically accumulates in a clumped fashion, which disrupts the appearance of normal nerve cells in the PD brain. The earliest stages of alpha-synuclein aggregation occur without forming Lewy bodies, but eventually, the final outcome of the highly aggregated forms of this protein is the Lewy body. These changes, although invisible to patients and their physicians, are the core features of PD at the cellular level, and they are the primary targets for therapies to prevent the development and progression of this disorder.

Stages of Parkinson's

The symptoms you experience with PD are brought about by specific changes in groups of nerve cells situated in the parts of the brain that govern movement. These paired structures (on the right and left sides of the brain) are called the *basal ganglia* (they are also known as the *striatum*). In PD, nerve cells in this region die off very slowly over many years, for unknown reasons. When 50 percent or more of this nerve cell population has been lost, symptoms emerge. Prior to reaching that threshold, even though thousands of nerve cells have been lost, no outward symptoms of PD emerge. Obviously, this phase of the illness would be an ideal time to start a protective therapy, if only this preclinical stage could be discerned. In any case, the progressive decline in remaining functional nerve cells eventually results in impaired signaling through the brain circuits that govern motor control, and the disorder becomes more obvious. Evidence of PD can simultaneously be evident in impaired dexterity and walking, as well as tremors. In summary, the earliest stages of PD occur at a basic cellular level that is undetectable, and at present we don't know when this stage (known as the prodromal period) starts. There is emerging evidence that, preceding these changes in the brain, similar changes happen in nerve cells in the muscle walls of the large intestine and possibly elsewhere in the body, but that research has yet to offer anything concrete about the earliest developments leading to the neurological aspects of PD. Unfortunately, since we're currently unable to detect the disease in the preclinical phase, we don't have the means to make such an early diagnosis, nor do we (yet) have treatments that are able to arrest further nerve cell loss. Achieving both these goals, early detection and early diagnosis, is presently the topic of tremendous research interest worldwide. Before long, we hope that it will be possible to intervene at this preclinical stage of PD and establish diagnosis and treatment.

Unlike for diseases such as cancer, there is no established system that has achieved consensus for categorizing developmental stages of PD. Some possible groupings come to mind—those with tremor, for example (about two-thirds of all patients), and those without it. It may seem counterintuitive, but having tremors actually indicates a reduced risk for progression to disabling PD compared to patients lacking tremors. Hence, this distinction has some relevance for prognosis. However, the progression of the disease (and specifically how quickly it might worsen) varies greatly from patient to patient. It is worth emphasizing that many patients demonstrate very little progression over the course of months or years. This may be in part because available medications are adept at masking PD symptoms, even though the disorder may be progressing underneath effective symptomatic treatment. As we'll learn later, medications only give symptomatic relief; they do not possess the ability to intervene in the disease's progression. A patient rarely knows what's going on in their brain or shows outward signs of disease progression unless their medications are intentionally reduced or discontinued. On occasion, a patient may reduce or discontinue use of their medications for a short time to discover how effective they are. Another way researchers gauge PD progression is a brain imaging test called the dopamine transporter scan (commercially available as the DaTscan). A DaTscan is used for measuring the loss of affected nerve cells in the part of the brain from which motor impairments arise. DaTscans involve administering a radioisotope tracer intravenously to test for PD in a study that takes about four hours. Although useful as a research tool, this test isn't needed in everyday clinical practice. DaTscans are unnecessary if a patient's current medications are effectively managing symptoms.

As you research PD, you might encounter a staging system called the Hoehn and Yahr (H&Y) rating. This scale, which was created in the 1960s before the development of today's effective medications, was used to classify PD patients by describing sequential clinical changes over time. Keep in mind that this scale was developed to categorize patients who were followed over many years in an unmedicated state—this was the era before levodopa (a medication used to treat PD). According to the H&Y scale, Stage 1 refers to a patient with PD symptoms that are entirely one-sided, while Stage 2 has bilateral (both sides) involvement. H&Y Stage 3 patients have an additional problem of imbalance. To test for imbalance, a clinician has a patient stand and pulls on their shoulders to cause a sudden backward displacement. Yanking the patient backward forces the patient to recover against falling by steps and trunk movements to avoid toppling backward. Stage 3 patients may require several steps to avoid a fall, or no protective response might occur. Not surprisingly, Stage 3 correlates with increased risk for falls, and patients usually don't acquire this type of imbalance for at least three years or longer, if ever. By five or more years after the diagnosis of PD, as many as one-third of patients might exhibit retropulsive imbalance in clinical testing, meaning they would be classified as Stage 3. As important a milestone as H&Y Stage 3 can be envisioned to be, this finding is not, by itself, a sign that a patient is losing the ability to walk independently. Rather, the finding of imbalance provides a warning that measures to prevent falls (like the use of a cane or a walker) may become important for future safety.

For several reasons, a staging scale like the H&Y rating isn't relevant today for understanding current and future problems posed by PD. For example, in the 1960s when the H&Y scale was developed, Stages 4 and 5 were defined as requiring the use of a wheelchair or being unable to leave bed, respectively. These problems would be seen in a significant number of patients today if we didn't have the effective medications now in routine use.

Through 1970, some patients described as Stages 4 and 5 had been afflicted with PD for more than 10 years, and all had gone untreated by effective medication. In the current era, a much smaller fraction of PD patients would be classified as H&Y Stage 4 or 5, because of today's effective treatments.

In my view, the best way to categorize PD patients is based on medication responsiveness. If patients respond well to the available therapies and are able to keep their symptoms under control consistently, they would be categorized as having a mild stage of the disease. Those lacking a favorable response to medication or other treatments would be categorized as having advanced disease. Other factors to consider in classifying or categorizing PD patients could be the impact of other health concerns, such as cognition and physical

Common Myths and Misconceptions

In the current body of knowledge about PD, no cause or causes have been identified. Hence, neither stress, lifestyle, diet, exercise, sleeping habits, vitamin deficiency, nor work exposures either increase or decrease one's risk of acquiring it (though see "Causes of Parkinson's" on page 15 for information on how exposure to certain chemicals or pesticides can increase the risk). With the current absence of knowledge about the cause or causes of PD, it is difficult to envision how someone might make a claim about how to cure or prevent PD. Nevertheless, treatments with such assertions are rampant on the Internet and at health food stores. There are also other information outlets that promote unverified or unscientific products as PD treatments; be wary of these, as at the moment, there is nothing known that even hints at a way to halt PD. Examples of these unverified "treatments" include glutathione intravenous injections, electromagnetic field mats, stem cell injections, and other far-fetched remedies that shamelessly exploit patients who are in search of the same thing that legitimate medical research also seeks: a cure. Place your trust in medical professionals, not the far reaches of the Internet, if you wish to learn about the latest options undergoing research for PD treatments. Consult authoritative neurologists, especially movement disorder specialists, for the best course of treatment in managing your symptoms.

Another common myth is that, over time, patients can become "immune" to levodopa (which is a commonly used medication to treat PD; we'll discuss this drug more in detail later) and other PD medications. During chronic PD therapy, there can be fluctuations in a patient's optimal dose of medications, and new symptoms can emerge or evolve over time. However, PD medications do not lose their overall effectiveness over the years after starting them, and PD patients do not need larger and larger doses. There are also no addictive properties of PD medications. Hence, there is no established reason to hold off on beginning treatment with levodopa or other medications. This provision holds for those patients whose symptoms are quite mild or intermittent or whose PD began at a young age.

conditioning, a very sedentary lifestyle, severe arthritis, and heart disease. These factors all have a significant impact on physical functioning independent of PD, and other brain disorders, such as Alzheimer's disease, can interfere with cognition independently of PD. Clinicians also consider patients in terms of their overall duration of PD. Factors such as age of onset and duration of symptoms are also important determinants of prognosis and disability. The main point here is that there is no established staging scheme that every PD patient passes through.

Not All Parkinsonism Is PD

As a brain disease, PD is distinctive in terms of what is going on at the cellular level. Unlike the situation in the living patient, the picture within the brain is easy to recognize with high certainty. Viewed under a microscope, samples of PD brain tissue present an unmistakable picture of what has gone wrong. These observations include the marked loss of nerve cells in specific brain regions, such as the upper region of the brain stem (the connection between the spinal cord and the larger brain structure). The scientific name of the small territory involved is the *substantia nigra pars compacta*. It is here where major accumulations of aggregated alpha-synuclein protein occupy surviving nerve cells. These aggregations form circular structures called Lewy bodies. Even though the warning signs, symptoms, and disease progression vary widely from patient to patient, the presence of Lewy bodies at characteristic sites in the brain tissue is something that all PD patients have in common. Other types of pathological nerve cell changes in brain tissue can produce symptoms resembling those observed in PD. Though these disorders share some overlapping symptoms with PD, these conditions can be clearly distinguished as entirely different forms of Parkinsonism.

Progressive supranuclear palsy (PSP) is one of the Parkinsonian disorders that can mimic PD. PSP is a disorder marked by slowed movements, changes in gait, imbalance, and other features common to patients with PD. However, a skilled clinician can usually distinguish PSP from PD through certain findings on a neurological examination and through additional testing (especially an MRI scan of the brain, which would be normal in PD). Nonetheless, making the distinction between PD and PSP sometimes can be challenging in the weeks and months after symptoms have become apparent. PSP is much less common in the general population than PD and just one of several neurodegenerative disorders that, like PD, also involve progressive loss of brain nerve cells and motor impairments. It is not hereditary or associated with environmental exposures, concomitant illnesses, or other clues to why it develops. Usually, there are several aspects of the patient's history and clinical exam that permit a neurologist or movement disorder specialist to recognize PSP and to make a diagnosis other than PD. In PSP, there is a characteristic change in a portion of the brain as seen on an MRI scan that has been described as the "hummingbird sign," which will sometimes help in the process of differentiating PSP from PD. Evaluating eye movements for distinctive abnormalities, testing for blood pressure drop upon standing, and examining for other neurological deficits can help identify other alternative Parkinsonian disorders, which tend to be less common than either PD or PSP. Among these additional conditions with features of PD are multiple system atrophy (MSA), corticobasal degeneration (CBD), and frontotemporal dementia (FTD). There are several other disorders, though most of them are extremely rare. In some instances, these other Parkinsonian disorders are genetic in origin and can begin much earlier in life than typical PD. In general, their manifestations only partially resemble typical presentations of PD. For example, two genetic disorders, Wilson's disease and Huntington's disease, most commonly present an entirely different set of signs and symptoms from PD. However, rare instances can present a clinical profile indistinguishable from PD and thereby pose a very difficult diagnostic challenge even for a highly skilled specialist.

One way a clinician can classify the differences between cases of PD has to do with the treatment options. How patients respond to medications is, of course, an important practical matter. Certain PD medications target tremors, while others have the capability to improve slowed movement, gait, and dexterity in addition to tremors. Some patients are faced with impaired balance and gait problems that might not respond to available medications but can be managed with nonmedication approaches to improving function. These include the use of a cane or a walker and being mindful of balance when walking backward and pivoting. Considering the broad range of impairments imposed by PD, I sometimes use a simplistic PD categorization of a particular patient's disorder as either "good" or "bad" for a global description of the disorder. "Good" means that with proper medications, exercise, a strong support system in place, and a little bit of luck and pluck, even a person who has spent years living with this disorder will never advance to a "bad" version. "Bad" problems with PD include medication intolerance, involuntary movements, or gait and balance problems so significant that safe ambulation is not possible.

Causes of Parkinson's

Over the past half century, there has been no shortage of research interest in the cause or causes of PD. The challenges for gaining insights into this problem are huge, since as noted in the sidebar (see page 10), no single lifestyle factor has been correlated with the development of the disease. (However, it should be noted that agricultural workers who have been exposed to various chemicals and pesticides have been shown to have an increased risk for developing PD.) Diet, something that can have a direct effect on so many other diseases and disorders, has no apparent influence on one's risk for acquiring PD or on changing its course. Curiously, cigarette smoking and caffeine intake have been shown in many epidemiological studies to lessen the risk of acquiring PD. Despite these observations, PD can still develop despite heavy intake of caffeine and lifelong smoking (and of course, we now know enough about cigarette smoking to know that any benefits it may provide in the reduction of the risk of PD are offset by its many health risks).

As previously noted, PD was first described by Dr. James Parkinson more than two centuries ago, so it would seem that a modern diet and everyday chemical exposures are unlikely to explain its origins. Today, PD can be found worldwide and in all human populations. It does not occur in any animals. It doesn't spread from person to person, and experimental inoculation of brain tissue from a PD sufferer does not transmit the disorder when implanted into the brain of an experimental animal. What we do know is that the major risk for PD is advancing age. Most cases do not arise until the patient is in their seventh decade. The average age of onset in several PD clinics has been found to be 58 years. The prevalence of PD increases further in older individuals, since its presence does not lessen longevity in patients who are receiving treatment. It's important to remember that people who develop PD are generally perfectly healthy. Males constitute about 60 percent of PD patients, but the reason for their increased risk is unknown.

For further reading, look to online organizations (such as those listed in the Resources section starting on page 108) for the latest information on what research is telling us about PD's origins. A hot topic of current research is the genetic side of PD, particularly aimed at the question of whether gene mutations factor into the risk for developing the disease. A tiny fraction of PD cases arise from certain genetic mutations that, for those families affected, lead to the disorder in a "dominant" fashion, meaning that 50 percent of offspring will develop the disorder. For the most part, however, gene mutations detected in the PD population merely confer increased risk and do not inevitably cause PD. Current hypotheses pertaining to enhanced-risk genes envision these "cooperating" with environmental or lifestyle factors to trigger the final common pathway in PD causation. Even with more than two dozen enhanced-risk genes currently identified, most cases of PD lack any of these. Currently, there isn't a compelling reason for a PD patient to undertake testing for the commercially available genetic testing options. Positive or negative results in searching for PD-associated genes will not yield information that would alter current treatment options, nor would they provide health information useful for the rest of the patient's family. In the future, treatments for PD might very well depend on knowledge of gene testing results for guiding the use of individualized therapies that might be developed.

The aging process is one of cumulative effects, which might explain the relatively late arrival of PD in the life of those affected. As one gets older, there is a continual loss of nerve cells in the brain (including those in the specific regions affected in PD). However, the brain also possesses a tremendous reserve of nerve cells, which is one plausible explanation for why most people will never develop PD even at an advanced age. Brain scientists have identified several clues to what might be happening in the initiation of PD, such as the activation of inflammatory mechanisms in the brain. Another process readily seen in the PD brain is the aggregation of the vulnerable protein alpha-synuclein, which forms a characteristic abnormality in nerve cells, the Lewy body. Because of the size that Lewy bodies can grow to, one thought is that they can obstruct vital cellular functions. Another possible disease mechanism is the formation of toxic cellular by-products called free radicals or excitotoxins, which can be damaging to nerve cells. Each of these mechanisms (and many others) has undergone extensive study in the PD brain and in animal models of Parkinsonism. Some of them have been used as the rationale for clinical trials attempting to halt disease progression through targeted pharmacological approaches, like blocking potentially toxic mechanisms. One example of clinical research investigating a possible disease mechanism is a large clinical trial in which the antioxidant alpha-tocopherol (vitamin E) was administered for up to two years at a high dose. While this vitamin is a necessary dietary component for maintaining good health, this research study conclusively proved that supplementation with alpha-tocopherol did not slow PD progression.

So far, and despite a great deal of careful thinking on the matter, no one mechanism stands out as the likely common pathway for causing PD. In fact, it is still uncertain whether the mechanism that first causes PD is necessarily the same mechanism behind its progression, though it does seem logical to link the two processes. We do know that all cases of PD share the common pathological changes mentioned on page 17—loss of nerve cells and the formation of Lewy bodies within them—but distinguishing between cause and effect are still muddled concepts in PD. Alpha-synuclein aggregation seems to be not just a "victim" of the disease processes in the causation of PD, but more likely a specific inciting factor, for reasons that have yet to be discerned.

Connected to the alpha-synuclein story is another exciting dimension of PD research that looks beyond the brain to another region of the body where the disease might start. Several findings point to the possibility that it might originate in the large intestine (colon). The bacterial environment of the colon has an extremely diverse collection of microorganisms during lifelong exposure. These bacteria are a necessary part of our digestive system, but the origins of PD may be lurking in some strains. Several directions of recent research implicate these microorganisms (the entire population is generally called the gut *microbiome*) as a possible early-stage cause of PD. Whether these findings will translate into a therapy or preventive strategy remains to be seen.

Researchers and physicians maintain a high level of optimism about a future cure or preventive strategy for PD. Several clinical trials are currently underway testing research ideas that have come from many research laboratories all over the world. In chapter 1, I hope you gained some insight into how the various clues that PD provides translate into research. In the next chapter, we'll delve into better understanding the symptoms and how to recognize them, and how to get a firm grasp on the diagnosis of PD and all that it entails.

CHAPTER 2
Making Sense of
Your Diagnosis

W e know now that PD can present itself in several ways, with a variety of symptoms. In this chapter, we'll delve deeper into the range of signs and symptoms that characterize this disorder. Not all of these signs and symptoms affect everyone—especially early on, as it's not uncommon to experience just one or two symptoms, such as tremors, trailing-off handwriting, or decreased arm swing that can affect only one side of the body. Even further on in the development of PD, symptoms can appear intermittently, such as a tremor appearing only when the affected person is in a stressful situation. For most people, the history of how symptoms developed and the physician's observation of them constitute the entire basis for diagnosis. Diagnoses can be made by both inclusion (highly suggestive findings, like, for example, handwriting that trails off or presence of tremors with the hand at rest) and exclusion (for example, if symptoms came on abruptly, or unexplained weakness or imbalance). Diagnostic markers (lab tests) indicate that PD does not show up in blood tests. Imaging of the brain by CT or MRI scans generally yields normal results in PD. Sometimes it is the history—a report that walking has become gradually slower in a formerly fast-paced person, for example—that most drives a physician's suspicion of PD, even in the absence of any overt abnormalities in the office examination. As mentioned earlier, a resting tremor doesn't have to be present; sometimes all that is experienced is an internal perception of tremor that is not outwardly seen. A curious feature of this subjective sensation of tremor is that it can respond to the same medications used for a witnessed tremor. As you've seen, it is sometimes challenging to correlate typical symptoms of Parkinsonism with a definite diagnosis of PD, especially since several other disorders share similar symptoms and warning signs. In the sections ahead we'll look more closely at PD's symptoms in their different forms.

Understanding Your Symptoms

If you've been diagnosed with PD, keep in mind that many physicians, particularly neurologists, should be familiar with this disorder. It's not that rare, and modern medical education always covers this topic. Difficulties in your everyday functioning that may be quite puzzling to you (such as downward clenching of toes in one foot, for example) may nonetheless correspond to well-known, "classic" features of PD. Then again, physicians have been known to be wrong from time to time.

Recent research has highlighted the challenging problem of PD misdiagnoses. There are many cases that have been studied for the unique situation of typical signs and symptoms in patients who lack positive results on one of the most sensitive diagnostic tests for PD. This test is a radioisotope hospital investigation called a DaTscan. In this test, the injected radioisotope is bound to a molecule that sticks to the same region of the brain where changes in nerve cells develop. All patients with PD should have abnormal DaTscan findings. However, as many as 15 percent of persons with tremors, slowed movements, decreased arm swing, and other typical PD features have normal DaTscans; hence, they can be proven *not* to have PD. One might think that obtaining the highest level of certainty about a PD diagnosis might be important; on this basis, should everyone undergo DaTscan testing? The answer is probably no, since there is no available cure for PD, and it isn't currently necessary to be 100 percent sure of a correct diagnosis.

MOTOR SYMPTOMS

Virtually all PD is diagnosed in persons with obvious motor signs, meaning that clinical findings observed by a physician upon examination and the patient's history fit the description of typical impairments associated with PD. Slowed, repetitive tapping of the fingers and feet are a common feature. It can be one-sided or present symmetrically on both sides. Slow rising from a chair or turning in bed is another clue to PD. Increased effort required and slowed performance at dexterity-demanding tasks such as buttoning a shirt, placing arms in sleeves, and using a knife and fork are typical. PD patients often explain these problems as "feeling weak." However, when a clinician formally tests for muscle power, the PD patient will generally show full strength; hence, muscle performance power isn't hindered in PD, and the perception of weakness can be attributed to the slowness PD imposes on certain activities. Nonetheless, there is often a report of excessive fatigue during everyday tasks, particularly those that are more physically demanding, like walking a dog or carrying grocery bags. PD patients often report the need for resting between physical activities, whereas previously they might not have needed such breaks.

The PD experience illustrates how much of an intrinsic motor repertoire all of us possess and how second nature so many of our daily movements are. For example, the agility of facial muscles in involuntary response to speech or even thinking can be compromised in a person with PD. Facial inexpressiveness in people with PD is subject to misinterpretation by others as sadness or indifference. The diminished blink rate can lead to a false impression that a patient is intentionally staring; the lips can be slightly parted, suggesting a vacant facial expression. Differences in speech in a person with PD also become more pronounced. Speech can seem diminished in volume, less distinct, or modulated in pitch, and it can sometimes trail off, as if the person forgets what they're saying midsentence. In PD, adventitious movements, such as arm swing during walking or synergies between trunk and leg muscles while turning, can be diminished. The overall impression of motor impairment, as one patient told me, can be described as moving through life "dipped in glue." Imagine moving through a swimming pool filled with pudding instead of water, and consider how slowed down all your movements would be. Dexterity characteristically declines after a few seconds as the task continues, frustrating the person who's trying to button a shirt or tie a shoelace. For handwriting, the size and clarity of continued writing tends to become smaller and slower in execution.

Tremors occurring in limbs (especially the fingers) and the lips can also herald PD's onset. For many patients, the only initial symptom is a tremor. Characteristically, the tremor exhibits extreme regularity, occurring only in limbs when they are at rest. Tremor goes away when the limb is in motion. Stressful situations can enhance it, making it more apparent and easier to recognize. It is important to keep in mind that in the general population, there are more common causes of tremor than PD. Among these are essential tremor, which is often hereditary, and tremor caused as a side effect of medication.

In a person with PD, a tendency for forward flexed trunk posture and other changes in posture may exist. Hands can take on a flexed, tented posture. Sometimes there is a slight tilt of the trunk to one side. Another postural change that can be experienced in early PD is an abnormal turning in of a foot or downward clenching of toes. This condition, called foot *dystonia*, can be painful due to tight muscle spasms. Foot dystonia can cause stumbling during walking.

We recognize the motor symptoms characteristic of PD, but it's equally important to emphasize what motor symptoms do not occur in PD. For example, this disorder does not cause paralysis of any muscle. Those muscles that carry out breathing and swallowing functions are not affected. Coordination is largely spared, as is balance for most patients. Other neurological functions such as sensation, vision, hearing, and thinking are not affected by PD. However, some patients partially or completely lose their sense of smell because of nerve cell changes that develop in regions of the brain with a class of nerve cells similar to those found in the region that controls movement. When I discuss what is amiss in PD, I like to emphasize the limited functions that are vulnerable to this disorder. You may experience

Managing Sleep Disruptions and Disordered Sleep

Disrupted and unsatisfying sleep are unfortunately common features of PD. In fact, for several years before the onset of tremors or other outward manifestations of this disorder, people who will go on to develop PD are often plagued by vivid dreaming. An excessive amount of time in a dreaming stage of sleep can be measured by an overnight sleep lab study, though it's important to note that this finding alone does not mean that a diagnosis of PD will always follow. During dreams, "acting out," like limb movements and talking, can persist, sometimes for hours. Abrupt movements can be violent enough to cause injuries. Intense and lengthy dreaming like this can lead to chronic sleep deprivation (since fitful dreaming is not the deep, restful sleep needed) and daytime drowsiness, even though a PD patient might not recall the dreams or being awakened during the night. In addition to vivid dreaming, downward cramping of the feet (dystonia) is another cause of sleep disruption in PD. Fortunately, medications are available that can usually solve problems with sleep disruptions and provide relief to a person living with PD.

tremors, and your sense of smell may decrease, but you won't go on to paralysis, and your breathing and swallowing are not compromised. In the face of a disease that can seem over-whelming at times, it's important to keep in mind the positives.

NONMOTOR SYMPTOMS

Nonmotor symptoms refer to characteristic features of PD that differ greatly from the symptoms and signs mentioned in the previous section. One example is an increased chance of experiencing constipation. This problem can precede by several years the onset of PD motor features. Constipation is one of the many discomforts linked to the total body involvement that PD seems to be capable of. There is nothing specifically known about PD-associated constipation or how it can be prevented or managed, though you can try drinking more water and eating more fiber, both of which are good things to do regardless of what's causing your constipation. Another example of a nonmotor PD symptom is the tendency for daytime drool-ing. Although it might seem attributable to excessive salivary gland output, the problem is actually due to the decreased rate of spontaneous swallowing that all of us do semiautomatically several times per minute. With constant saliva production not met by an adequate rate of swallowing, the effect is the pooling of saliva, which causes drooling.

Some other nonmotor symptoms of PD, such as sleep and mood disorders, are discussed elsewhere in this chapter. Early on, some patients experience deep aches or sensations of hot or cold in their limbs as sensory features of PD. Clinicians should be familiar with the scope of nonmotor features, but for the patient, it's important to understand that not every discomfort or problem experienced is necessarily due to PD. A person with

PD can also have problems with diabetes, low thyroid hormone levels, aching joints, and a host of other nuisances and changes that are not necessarily correlated with PD but are simply part of the territory of getting older and our bodies aging.

Parkinson's Effects on the Brain

As we've learned, PD is primarily an affliction of the brain. Even if it originates elsewhere in the body, such as in the large intestine, the brain is the ultimate target of the disease. Slow muscle movement, decreased dexterity, and tremors reflect the impaired pattern of instructions dispatched by nerve cells in the brain. The hallmark of PD, which explains why movement is slowed and otherwise impaired, is the loss of a particular group of nerve cells that connect to the part of the brain called the striatum. These nerve cells release a signaling chemical called dopamine that activates circuitry so that movement happens. As the disease develops, nerve cells are lost, leading to diminished movement. Since most people diagnosed with PD already have greatly diminished stores of this chemical system, physicians commonly employ a strategy of replacement therapy. The approach leads to some of the most dramatic medication effects that can be observed in all of medical therapeutics. Dopamine replacement therapy, developed in the late 1960s, reverses the deficiency of dopamine in the striatum, and it is still considered to be the most effective way to treat PD. When dopamine signaling in the striatum is restored, virtually all motor impairment symptoms of PD can be reversed in response to the normalization of brain circuitry.

In practice, however, managing PD treatment is much more complicated than simply restoring dopamine. For instance, PD tremors seem to involve circuits and signaling chemicals different from those using dopamine. On this basis, medications effective against PD tremors may act independently of dopamine-mediated signaling. Of course, the biggest mystery is why this all happens in the first place. The loss of a discrete group of nerve cells—several hundred thousand at most, and with their adjacent neighbors spared—is what challenges researchers to find out what is unique in the metabolism, structure, and function of the various nerve cell groups lost in PD. Other nerve cell groups elsewhere in the brain, like those in the olfactory region (which governs the sense of smell), also die out to some extent, which is the reason some PD patients suffer from loss or reduction of their sense of smell. Not all the affected nerve cell groups utilize dopamine, which adds another layer of complexity, since there are other brain chemicals at play. However, every PD brain shows the presence of the masses of alpha-synuclein proteins that form Lewy bodies. Thus, in order to answer the mystery of why PD occurs, we first need to answer the mystery of why these Lewy bodies develop.

The PD brain has been studied extensively for the possibility that the cause of PD might be detectable in microscopic or biochemical analyses. These types of inquiry have been informative, though neither has provided a definitive answer. One promising direction of research has led to the recognition of several regional biochemical abnormalities. In some nerve cells there is diminished enzymatic generation of an important antioxidant in the brain called glutathione. When glutathione encounters a free radical (a chemical compound that can be toxic to nerve cells), it squashes its toxic activity to render it harmless. Another finding of interest with regard to PD causation has to do with inflammatory processes, which refer to the activation of chemical systems in the body that protect us from infections and initiate wound healing, among other functions. There is strong evidence that various inflammatory responses are chronically unregulated in the PD brain, suggesting some inciting trigger. Other research has investigated whether trace minerals in the PD brain differ from those in healthy brains. For example, PD brains show evidence for increased deposits of iron in the groups of nerve cells that are affected in PD. The increased concentrations of iron fit into a hypothesis of increased vulnerability of these cells to toxicity from free radicals. Mitochondria (the energy units of all cells) have been found in PD to possess a metabolic abnormality in the brain and throughout the body. Finally, patterns of cell-to-cell communication through nerve circuits in the PD brain show distinctly different findings from those of healthy individuals. These patterns, detected with a brain imaging technique called a PET scan, may offer a useful biomarker, or diagnostic tool, that could be used to establish an early diagnosis or proof of treatment efficacy.

Can I Slow Down My PD?

While the cause or causes of PD remain unknown, it seems possible that in the future, it may be possible to arrest the disease's progression. Current research is focused on this goal. However, at present, there just isn't any solid information that can guide a patient toward this goal. Many therapeutic approaches and interventions have shown promise in the laboratory, such as vitamin E, coenzyme Q10, and other antioxidant and anti-inflammatory approaches. However, when tested in clinical trials, they did not lead to success. So far, no dietary or medication influences have definitively shown an ability to slow down the progression of PD.

One example of how this research is proceeding is the recent experience with a compound used to artificially elevate uric acid concentrations throughout the body. Uric acid is a natural antioxidant, and several epidemiological studies have shown that the higher the concentration of uric acid in the blood, the lower the risk for acquiring PD. (The rate of the disease's progression was also shown to be slower with higher concentrations of uric acid in the blood.) However, the large-scale clinical trial of this hypothesis was unfortunately not rewarded with evidence for disease modification. Even though the study showed a correlation between higher blood concentrations of uric acid and fewer instances of PD, that correlation did not necessarily prove the existence of a factor that caused PD or enhanced its progression; in this case, correlation did not necessarily imply causation. As it happens, much clinical research has to proceed on the basis of nothing more than an educated hunch, and PD presents the same challenges for progress in research.

At present, the best advice for warding off PD and other diseases is to stay healthy overall, exercise regularly, and eat a balanced, healthy diet. There is some intriguing evidence from animal studies that endurance training and some other types of exercise may exert an influence on the PD brain that could slow the rate of disease progression. Even if this strategy doesn't work, the effects of exercise can only impart positive health benefits for someone with PD. There is no current evidence that any

Dealing with Depression
and Anxiety

In the general population, depression and anxiety are not rare occurrences. According to the World Health Organization, depression and anxiety disorder affect more than 264 million people and 300 million people worldwide, respectively. For those living with PD, depression and anxiety somewhat increase in prevalence. The strain of living with a chronic ailment and the accompanying difficulties likely contribute to a greater risk for depression and anxiety. However, evidence for increased risk of depression even before the onset of outward PD symptoms has also been found. Perhaps this increased propensity for depression has to do with biochemical changes in PD similar to those in the movement centers of the brain, but there's no information that definitively proves that. Depression and anxiety symptoms can also appear commingled with the features of PD, such as diminished facial expression or tremulousness. For this reason, it is important for a physician to specifically inquire about a patient's mental health in order to advise on medications and treatments that can help. Many of the symptoms of PD overlap with those experienced by someone with depression. Effective medications are available that can help alleviate both anxiety and depression, and both issues have nonpharmaceutical approaches that may be considered as well. Medications used to treat depression or anxiety do not interfere with the symptomatic control of PD.

medications should be avoided in order to slow progression. A few drugs, including those used as tranquilizers and for gastrointestinal disorders, are well known to unmask or exacerbate the symptoms of PD. However, these effects are reversible and have nothing to do with the mechanisms of what causes PD.

Hope for a Cure

For a disorder carrying the threat of progressive disability like PD, a cure would seem to be far more desirable than simply masking its symptoms. Current research that focuses on improving symptomatic therapies does not go on at the expense of searching for the origins of PD or finding definitive treatments to cure it. However, researchers face certain basic challenges in the pursuit of a cure. By the time of diagnosis, PD is already at an advanced stage in the affected neuronal circuits of the brain. More than 60 percent of nerve cells are lost, and the remaining nerve cells might not be in good health or capable of optimal functioning. The goal of preventing PD requires diagnosis to be accomplished at the preclinical stage. Presently, diagnosis at this stage is not possible, even though a patient can spend years in this stage before any outward manifestations of the disease become apparent. Research into PD biomarkers is attempting to achieve a much earlier diagnosis so that the curative therapies of the future can be implemented early. Despite all of this, more than two dozen clinical trials have been conducted over the last 30 years with the goal of disease modification in mind. Disease modification implies the slowing or halting of the disease as measured by various PD rating scales gauging severity of tremors, slowed movement, handwriting changes, and several other symptoms. Many of these trials have taken place over the course of several years and have involved hundreds of patients. None has found a potential cure. Inadequate study methodologies, limited ability to model PD in animal experiments, and the possibility of multiple causes for PD may explain the lack of success so far. However, from the many efforts at finding a cure, a great deal of information has emerged that has helped guide subsequent studies. Improved understanding of the disease and the best ways to track its progression have been positive results of these clinical trials. Studies that failed to yield useful results have redirected the targets of clinical research to more promising topics. Over the past 30 years, clinical research carried out to achieve disease modification has received tremendous support from the pharmaceutical industry, government agencies like the National Institutes of Health, and patient advocacy organizations working with academic consortia like the Parkinson Study Group. Research findings are widely shared in publications, and international meetings are held annually by a huge community of dedicated researchers and scientists. For those of us who conduct PD research, we have reason to hope that finding a way to slow or halt further progression of the disease seems less a question of "if" than "when."

Hence, an optimistic perspective is well justified. The scientific research community has enthusiastically embraced the search for how to slow or stop PD. Modern laboratory science has made strong gains in mirroring the human disease in various models to explore causes and treatments. The translation of today's findings in a genetically modified roundworm or even a yeast cell into tomorrow's next medication trial has become a routine endeavor. If you're interested in learning more about the current research, the international course of PD clinical trials can be followed on the authoritative website ClinicalTrials.gov, and the various PD advocacy organizations listed in the Resources section (see page 108) also publicize this information.

In this chapter we've covered some key tools for understanding PD symptoms and getting a firm grasp on a PD diagnosis. The manifestations of PD can present in several different possible ways with varying severity of symptoms, and it's important to keep in mind that yours can be quite different from those of others with the same diagnosis. Although we are not yet able to slow or halt the progression of PD, current research is actively seeking treatments based on the many valuable clues we do have about the PD brain.

CHAPTER 3
Treating Your PD

In this chapter, we'll discuss the many forms of treatment for PD. Although understanding the biology of PD causation is still in the research phase, we nonetheless have a solid understanding of how to live with it. There is no standard regimen of care, since treatment is based on each person's symptoms. However, most PD patients have many components in common, including the use of a relatively standard medication called levodopa and the need to identify care providers. Not all cases of PD are managed in the same way; your choices for optimizing life with this disorder can go far beyond the medications you take. As we'll discuss in this chapter, a care team supporting you is an important strategy for making the most of your life with PD.

Assembling Your Care Team

When you or a loved one is newly diagnosed with PD, chances are you will be introduced to a cast of physicians and other health care professionals. Contact with a single physician (likely your primary doctor) might be the only relationship initiated by first seeking a diagnosis of PD, but some patients may choose to engage a broader care team to help them navigate and deal with the full impact of this disorder. In this section, we'll discuss the different roles of care providers you may encounter in your journey. Not every patient needs the full range of services that different medical professionals provide; however, this overview will showcase the options patients and their families can turn to for optimizing quality of life with PD.

PRIMARY CARE PROVIDER

Although PD is a neurological disorder, most patients receive regular medical attention from a primary care provider (PCP). Sometimes designated as a family physician or general practitioner, a PCP is often the first medical professional with whom one interacts when discussing new symptoms, managing commonplace medical complaints, and seeking out specialty advice. Most important, the PCP is often the first line of communication and comfort for all the ills of life. A PCP always has a medical degree, whether it's as a doctor of medicine (MD) or as a doctor of osteopathy (DO). Training as a chiropractor, homeopath, or naturopath does not provide the necessary qualifications to serve as a PCP in the diagnosis or treatment of PD. Depending on the health care system and location, PCPs are sometimes the only medical resources for people with PD, making them all the more critical as both your first line of defense and also your only designated medical professional. And sometimes access to PCPs can be so limited in a given practice that nurse practitioners (NPs) or physician assistants (PAs) provide the majority of the contact the patient will have with their medical professional. Nurse practitioners and physician assistants are highly trained clinicians whose roles are thought of as "team players" for the physicians they serve. In my experience, these "physician extenders" or "midlevels" (as the medical system sometimes terms them) can offer competent, quality care for neurological conditions like PD. Although a patient newly experiencing the signs and symptoms of PD might wish to seek out the highest level of clinical expertise, the next steps beyond diagnosis and initiation of treatment will often involve a PCP and his or her staff, which likely includes NPs and PAs.

A PCP is often the first person to discern the earliest inklings of PD. Even without the extensive neurological training possessed by a neurologist, a general medical education should be sufficient background for a PCP to suspect or even be certain of a PD diagnosis. Differentiating PD from other possible causes of tremor or gait impairment should be part of a PCP's skill set. A PCP should be familiar with medications commonly used to treat PD, especially their benefits, possible side effects, and potential interactions with any other medications a patient is currently taking. Many PCPs whose patient population includes older individuals might have greater exposure to PD and, hence, more experience with management strategies. It is also important for people with PD to recognize that "general practitioners" have a broad range of patients coming in through the waiting room and not a great deal of time to devote to learning about the latest in PD information for physicians. Hence, it's possible that new developments in PD and experience in dealing with some of the complexities of the disorder may be outside the realm of a PCP's expertise or difficult for them to keep up with. Most experienced PCPs recognize their limits in managing a neurological disorder like PD and therefore might choose to refer a PD patient to a neurological physician rather than carrying out an evaluation by themselves.

The expectations of people with PD can be (rightfully so) quite high regarding the knowledge and capabilities of a trusted PCP. Deciding if and when to seek a second opinion or specialty advice can be a challenge. I can't speak for all medical professionals, but neurologists and, particularly, movement disorder specialists generally welcome consultations with PD patients to help provide the answers they seek and add their specialized expertise in education and decision-making for patients living with this disorder.

INTERNIST

An internist is a specialist in medical practice (generally this domain of medicine is called "internal medicine") whose training and certification is more extensive than that of most general practitioners, both in the intensity of training and in the number of years. The precise boundary between a PCP and an internist may be difficult to define. For many people, an internist can serve in the role of a PCP. However, internists generally limit their practice to a range of medical disorders involving the heart, GI tract, internal organs, joints, and other specific conditions whose diagnosis and management may go beyond the capabilities of a PCP. Furthermore, internists who have extra training and expertise work in the subspecialties of cardiology, gastroenterology, renal disease, and several other specified areas. Some internists have extra training and certification in the specialty of geriatrics. Internists also generally undergo more extensive training in neurology than that required for a PCP after medical school.

Given that the typical age at which PD is diagnosed skews toward the older years, it is likely that there will be another physician involved in the patient's overall health care maintenance team or previously consulted for treatment of some other medical condition. Partnership between an internist and a PCP in managing high blood pressure (hypertension), for example, is quite common. In my experience as a neurologist managing PD, I often share medical management responsibilities with internists or PCPs for my patients' common problems like constipation, low blood pressure symptoms (called postural hypotension), and sleep disorders. Communication within the care team of physicians is critical, because medications prescribed by one practitioner may have implications for what the other physician is trying to accomplish. For example, the start of a medication for PD can sometimes cause the lowering of blood pressure, changing the need for an antihypertension drug.

Physicians who have less expertise in diagnosing and managing PD can also learn valuable information from a neurological consultation. Patients seeking out a second opinion from a more specialized clinician like a neurologist or movement disorder specialist shouldn't fear a negative reaction from their internist or PCP. Seeking a second opinion does not indicate a loss of confidence in or urge to abandon the care of their usual physician. Most sensible physicians encourage referrals for a second opinion if a patient needs a boost in confidence, information, or, in some instances, competence in managing their disorder. This can be true even for patients with a mild version of PD.

Patient Advocacy Tips and FAQs

One of the most important things you can do as a PD patient is advocate for yourself and your care. This means asking your physician(s) the right questions and getting satisfactory answers. Some of these questions might include:

- How sure are you about my diagnosis (and do I have any other neurological problems)?
- Are there any new treatment options that I should be aware of?
- Do you want to hear back from me (by phone or email) after medication changes have been made?
- Based on my history and neurological exam, do I need brain imaging to be sure of my diagnosis?

Another important component of care and managing your condition is getting adequate support. Depending on where you live, there may be a local support group for PD. Over recent decades, support groups have sprung up independently or under the direction of several regional and national PD organizations. What is the support they offer, and why should you consider participating? The discussions at such meetings are often guided by experts who provide critical information on what is known currently about PD as well as what's new in PD research. Some areas have an array of specialized meetings, such as ones targeted to patients with young-onset PD or caregivers for those living with PD. If you're unable to attend a meeting in person or if your schedule doesn't allow it, seek out meetings that have an option to call in or video chat.

A newly diagnosed PD patient can learn a lot of practical information at these meetings. The concept of a support group may seem like an intimidating experience to some, and it can be challenging to publicly share one's private experience of living with PD or of a loved one living with it. My suggestion is to consider attending a support group once or twice as an experiment so that you can be open to its potential benefits. What you will see and hear may not necessarily duplicate your experience with PD. However, gaining the perspectives of other people living with this disorder can be extremely useful in getting a broader picture of the human impact of PD. There is also a good chance that participating in such a group will provide information that you may not otherwise get from your physician or through your own research reading books and blogs about PD (many of which are listed in the Resources section starting on page 108). For example, persons with PD have gotten excellent word-of-mouth advice on the best practitioners and resources in the community (physicians, physical therapists, pharmacists, exercise classes, and so on). Perhaps the biggest benefit to attending a support group is simply camaraderie with others dealing with PD or, if you're a caregiver, in other caregivers who are going through a similar experience. When you're facing a serious condition, knowing you're not alone in the fight is a beneficial perspective.

NEUROLOGIST

Seeking out a neurologist is a logical choice for most people who suspect a PD diagnosis or who have been recently diagnosed. A neurologist is an MD or DO who has completed four years of specialized residency training in a nationally approved program following medical school graduation. In addition to this training, a board-certified neurologist needs to pass difficult examinations to show competency in the practice of neurology. To maintain such certification, neurologists are required to continue medical education courses and, in some instances, undergo repeated examinations in neurology at several intervals throughout their careers. Diagnosis and management of PD is a core competency requirement of every neurologist's practice. Therefore, every neurologist should be regarded as a PD specialist. Some neurologists advertise their services as such. There is another category of neurologists, however, who have engaged in extra training beyond the four-year neurological training regimen in order to be designated as a movement disorder specialist (or subspecialist). This distinction does not come with board certification, however, since no organization has been established (so far) to assess competency in this subspecialty. Those neurologists who indicate that they are PD or movement disorder specialists have devoted one or more years of extra training to gain experience and expertise in this specialty. Several training centers in the United States and around the world provide this additional training, often at institutions where PD research is carried out and services for neurosurgical treatment of PD are provided. Many movement disorder specialists practice in academic settings that provide ongoing training for newly minted physicians and nurses as well as medical students.

Do you need to see a PD or movement disorder specialist? If the question is based on the likelihood of receiving optimal care, the answer is probably no. All physicians should have the skills to carry out a neurological examination and to weigh the evidence for establishing the diagnosis of PD. All physicians can prescribe PD medications, though depending on how much experience they have treating patients with PD, some might feel uncomfortable prescribing some PD drugs with which they have not become familiar, such as dopaminergic agonists (which we will discuss later in chapter 3); these drugs behave like the chemical dopamine that's deficient in PD and can have a number of possible side effects. The number of PD patients a neurologist sees can vary from practitioner to practitioner; even very busy neurologists may have in their patient mix only a small fraction of persons with PD. As a result, subspecialists such as movement disorder specialists may have more experience and knowledge about PD than neurologists who see fewer cases. It is difficult to generalize about whether every PD patient will benefit from seeking out a movement disorder clinician; they may offer the same information and treatment options as those provided by a general neurologist. However, a movement disorder specialist (I am one of these subspecialists, with three years of training in movement disorders after my neurology residency) should be expected to provide the highest level of advice and information about a broad range of PD topics, symptoms, and treatments. Many subspecialists in movement disorders routinely attend meetings and seminars specific to PD and closely keep up with the extensive medical research that is expanding our boundaries of knowledge about this disorder. As mentioned, many movement disorder specialists are involved in academic activities, including clinical research. On this basis, patients seeking out consultations with movement disorder specialists might be offered access to clinical trials of new therapies for PD. So, what would be your decision on this matter? Key questions to ask are 1) Are you satisfied with the quality of information provided by your physician (and do they answer your questions in a satisfactory manner)? and 2) Are your symptoms well controlled with your current treatment regimen? If the answers are yes, seeking a second opinion from a movement disorder specialist might not add any extra value.

SPEECH, PHYSICAL, AND OCCUPATIONAL THERAPISTS

Beyond the care provided by physicians, other health care professionals can offer PD patients specific forms of therapy with great benefits beyond those offered by medications alone. These therapies focus on the various challenges of daily life imposed by PD, such as voice problems (soft or trailing-off speech), gait impairment, and clumsiness. Speech, physical, and occupational therapy all bring to patients the specialized skills of highly trained and certified therapists who often have doctoral degrees. These specialties work with evidence-based strategies of directed training and structured plans for exercises to be practiced.

A speech therapist helps a patient achieve increased loudness, clarity, and ease of speech. Spoken communication is one of the most common problems I encounter, even among persons with otherwise mild PD. If you've never experienced difficulty with speech, these things may seem fairly simple to solve, but the road to improvement is almost always more complicated than it might seem. Speech therapy has been especially effective in the context of Lee Silverman Voice Treatment LOUD

(LSVT-LOUD), a program comprised of structured treatment sessions that are carried out over several weeks. The consortium that created and trains therapists for the specialized LSVT-LOUD speech therapy program has also created another training system that targets mobility problems of PD. This program is named LSVT-BIG and is a physical therapy program that tackles several common physical problems of PD, such as risk for falls, gait "freezing," difficulty in arising, and other disabilities that can be poorly controlled by medications. Another group of health professionals, occupational therapists, takes on the agenda of improving motor skills that can interfere with the execution of daily activities such as writing and dressing. Of course, the need for enlisting in one or more of these specialized therapy programs is highly individualized; in most cases, they are not needed by patients at the initial onset of PD (and many PD patients will never require them). If there are questions about what could be accomplished, a consultation session with one of these therapists can guide a patient's decision as to whether to begin one of these therapy regimens. It is worth noting that, for most patients with relatively mild PD symptoms, the greatest improvements will come from medications alone. Mild Parkinsonism generally doesn't necessitate the input of a speech, physical, or occupational therapist.

PSYCHOLOGIST

A psychologist is a licensed professional (often with doctoral training) whose professional abilities provide several benefits pertinent to the PD patient. Psychologists have the education and experience to evaluate possible problems like depression, maladaptive behaviors, and cognitive decline. As therapists, some psychologists also practice counseling and other types of psychotherapy.

Especially if equipped with knowledge about the disorder, a psychologist can provide services that are extremely beneficial to a PD patient. In most communities there should be a psychologist who is very familiar with PD. (One of my patients with PD serves in this role.) Social and personal well-being in living with PD is the theme of the services offered by psychologists. These services can be augmented with types of support also provided by psychiatrists, social workers, clergy, and even skilled PD support group leaders.

The professional competence of a licensed psychologist is more than just a college education in psychology and years of additional training; often, a psychologist holds a special and unique place in the life of someone with PD, offering nonjudgmental and supportive counseling that might not be readily available any other way. Psychologists vary greatly in their background, experience, and approach to helping. Finding the right psychologist might involve trial interviews or brief consultations, along with setting goals in the first one or two sessions before committing to a long-term therapeutic relationship. The PD patient might seek out psychological counseling if they wish to explore nonmedication approaches to solving problems like depression and anxiety. The goals of psychological care include improving coping skills and relaxation techniques, treating depression and anxiety, meeting in a structured way to share experiences and support, and being a regular, uncritical source for professional advice and support both in daily life and in crises.

NUTRITIONIST

The job of a nutritionist can mean several different things. A registered dietitian (abbreviated as RD) is one of them. An RD is a licensed health professional (often based in or employed by a hospital) who has an extensive education in nutrition and expertise in advising patients with various medical problems. A consultation with an RD can offer evidence-based dietary information. Nutritionists can provide ideas for healthy menus, strategies for weight loss, and the latest information on the compatibility of protein intake with PD medication, which we'll discuss more in the next part of the chapter. Information about diet and nutrition might also come from others who claim to be nutritionists, although not everyone offering such advice is nec-essarily qualified to dispense scientifically accurate information.

There are many opinions on what constitutes a healthy diet, and there are dozens of ways to accomplish this goal. However, in order to be entitled to take on such a trusted advisory role, a nutritionist should, above all, trust science and proven medical findings first. Nutritionists should not let unsubstantiated information creep into their counseling, such as the use of high-dose vitamins or nutritional supplements. There is actu-ally no recommended PD diet; no dietary regimen has been shown to have any influence on the risk for acquiring PD or the course of its progression. Many practitioners have earned the title of "nutritionist" through accredited schooling and scientifically guided training. Others who use the title take a more philosophical perspective, such as recommending diets limited to "natural" or "organic" foods or avoiding meat and processed foods. My suggestion regarding nutritional information is to be cautious in taking advice, even the well-meaning type, and if you seek the counsel of a nutritionist, make sure that you are satisfied with the nutritionist's qualifications and the message you hear.

SOCIAL WORKER

Social workers are professionals who are responsible for helping individuals, families, and groups of people cope with problems they're facing in an effort to enhance social functioning and well-being and generally improve the lives of their clients. Often, social workers are just the right professionals needed to facilitate sometimes-difficult adjustments for someone newly diagnosed with PD. For some people, the diagnosis alone can be a burden in adjusting to the new challenges ahead, especially within the family structure. For example, a patient new to PD may wish to seek out among family members or friends someone to take on a caregiver role. Discussions and decisions on how to make this happen can be facilitated by counseling meetings with a social worker. Some people with PD undergo stressful changes in lifestyle because of emerging disabilities, changes in employment, and the like; social workers can provide emotional support and useful guidance for how to network with and take advantage of a community's resources. In some ways, working with a social worker can be part of a continuum that links physicians, PD support groups, psychologists, family members, and other persons interested in the overall emotional health of a person with PD. Social workers must acquire extensive training and experience before they can be licensed to practice this profession.

As we've learned in this section, there is no standard treatment or therapy regimen for PD. The best course of treatment and medication will be tailored to the patient's symptoms and monitored regularly by their physician. Depending on the patient's needs, their care team may include a neurologist, a movement disorder specialist, and other health care professionals such as physical or speech therapists, psychologists, or social workers. It's important to be educated on the different providers available to persons living with PD so that they can make the best and most informed decisions for their individual needs and lifestyle.

Medications

The late 1960s heralded the modern era of PD, signaling a major change in what we know about the disease and how we treat it compared to the time of Dr. James Parkinson two centuries ago and his discovery of "the shaking palsy." Today, effective control of PD signs and symptoms can be achieved for most people. The most effective medications are affordable, and the pricier ones generally have generic equivalents that deliver equal results. For many patients, the side effects of medications are a minor problem, if they are perceived at all. Unfortunately, not all PD problems are alleviated by medications. The most glaring challenge is finding a treatment for slowing down the progression of the disease or preventing PD altogether. Nevertheless, even masking PD symptoms is enough for many patients to regard current therapies as sufficient for leading a near-normal life on a prolonged basis.

HELPFUL MEDICATIONS FOR THE NEWLY DIAGNOSED

A major theme of PD therapeutics is replacing a deficiency of signaling between nerve cells in a region of the brain (previously described as the striatum) that controls movement functions. As we learned in chapter 1, the missing chemical in the PD brain responsible for causing symptoms is a neurotransmitter substance called dopamine. Replacing dopamine-mediated signaling can be achieved in several ways. The earliest development is still the mainstay of current therapy: an amino acid called dihydroxy-L-phenylalanine (commonly called levodopa, abbreviated as L-DOPA). Levodopa occurs naturally in legume vegetables, such as certain beans, peas, and lentils. For medicinal purposes, levodopa is taken in larger quantities than food portions would provide. Levodopa is combined with another medicine, either carbidopa or benserazide, in a drug class called decarboxylase inhibitors. Ingested orally, levodopa is absorbed only in the upper portion of the small intestine. Once taken up by the same mechanism that absorbs nutrients, it reaches the bloodstream and eventually is passed into the brain, where it is converted to dopamine. The whole process requires at least 15 to 20 minutes at its fastest and can be more delayed at times.

Even the first dose of levodopa can produce a dramatic reversal of Parkinsonian symptomatology, albeit only temporarily. For the past half century since it was first developed, levodopa has been regarded as the "gold standard" treatment for PD. It is remarkably cost-effective, and it has allowed millions of patients living with PD to control their symptoms despite progression of the underlying disorder. Levodopa can have side effects in some persons, but it is generally a satisfactory treatment that never loses its efficacy. Extensive research has clarified many past controversies about levodopa. For example, a myth about the drug continues to circulate on the Internet that, after a few years, levodopa will decline in effectiveness or will always lead to the side effect of involuntary movements (dyskinesias). Neither of these suppositions has been supported by careful study. Today, we know that there are no reasons to avoid starting therapy with levodopa even for the mildest symptoms of PD.

For the newly diagnosed patient, levodopa plus a decarboxylase inhibitor (in the United States, carbidopa) is usually sufficient for controlling most symptoms of PD. In the United States and elsewhere, the brand name of the combination product is Sinemet. Today, only generic formulations of Sinemet are used, the most common one being carbidopa-levodopa 25-100 (reflecting the milligram content of each of the two combined ingredients). For many patients, one tablet taken three times daily at mealtimes is sufficient for maximal relief. Use of the 10-100 formulation is not recommended, and although there is also a 25-250 formulation, this dosage is generally more than the newly diagnosed patient needs. Carbidopa-levodopa is extremely safe and needs no blood test monitoring, nor does it cause any possible damage to internal organs. Levodopa also has virtually no dangerous interactions with other drugs. Its side effects, if experienced at all, are usually quite benign. Occasionally at the start of taking levodopa, a patient might experience nausea, vomiting, or light-headedness or faintness upon standing. Other side effects are possible but not common. For this drug and other medications you use, you should always check with your prescribing physician or pharmacist if you have any concerns about your PD medications.

Levodopa is the most commonly used medication for treating PD, but other drug therapies are also quite effective in some situations. They can be safely prescribed in conjunction with levodopa and taken at the same time. Of these options, the most commonly used are the two types of drugs that target resting tremors (which, it should be noted, don't always respond well or at all to levodopa). These drugs, called anticholinergics and amantadine, have been used as antitremor treatments for several decades. Among the anticholinergic drugs, the most used ones are trihexyphenidyl and benztropine. Each of these is a generic drug. They are generally well-tolerated adjuncts to levodopa.

Another treatment option for PD symptoms, though rarely used in newly diagnosed cases, is a class of drugs called dopaminergic agonists. These drugs include pramipexole, ropinirole, and rotigotine. The first two are ingested orally, and rotigotine is administered through the skin in a patch form. As a group, the dopaminergic agonists mimic the actions of dopamine in the PD brain. They could be used as alternatives to levodopa, but there is no demonstrated reason to do so, since they are more expensive and potentially can cause more side effects. Dopaminergic agonists do have an important role in therapy for certain PD problems that typically can evolve several years into the disorder. Their usefulness is based in part on their longer duration of action. Examples of their usefulness include actions on painful muscle cramping of the feet at night and tremors not responsive to other medication options. This class of drugs is also effective for treating another common neurological disorder called restless-leg syndrome, in which the incessant and uncomfortable urge to move the legs at night can make sleeping difficult.

KEEPING TRACK OF MEDICATIONS

Just like therapies and treatment regimens, medications for PD are not used in identical fashion for every patient. There are, however, some general principles that are abided by for most patients. As mentioned in the previous section, levodopa is the backbone therapy onto which other treatments can be added if needed—for example, to block involuntary movements caused by levodopa or to halt tremors uncontrolled by levodopa adjustments. The problems of multiple daily doses of levodopa can be compounded by a medication schedule that incorporates other drugs at various times throughout the day, since each drug has different rules for optimal use. For example, many patients find the ideal spacing of levodopa to be three or four hours between doses after a few years, whereas amantadine doses are continually effective for six or more hours. Some PD drugs are effective with once-daily dosing. Keeping track of a multi-medication (polypharmacy) approach to PD can be challenging. Staying on top of medications can call for extra attention in this era of generic formulations, since the appearance (shape, color, size) of generic pills might change from refill to refill, as there is often more than one generic drug manufacturer for the same prescription. Carbidopa-levodopa 25-100 (the most commonly used form of levodopa) is color-coded such that it is always yellow (varying in shade, though), but its pill shape can vary from round to oval. Many patients also struggle not only with the problem of missing doses during the day but also with the problem of potentially doubling doses when failing to recall that a dose was already swallowed. Perhaps the best strategy for avoiding both problems is a container consisting of multiple compartments in which you can line up the day's regimen of pills. You can find many useful compartmented containers of this type in your local drugstore or for purchase online. Keep in mind that since medications for PD do not aim to cure (since there is no cure), they are only for symptomatic therapy, and a missed dose doesn't have any consequences other than temporarily diminished benefit to the patient.

Experimental Treatments

PD is unique in the vast number of clinical trials undertaken over the past 60 years seeking better treatments. Among these are treatments that have been tested to learn whether they could halt progression or even cure the disease. Starting with the development of anticholinergic drugs in the 1950s, there have been dozens of other new drugs tested in patients in clinical trials, culminating in the development and current use of seven classes of drugs. Many other tested drugs have fallen out of use because of inefficacy, unacceptable side effects, or other undesirable factors. The theme of most PD clinical therapeutics research has been primarily the discovery of drugs that are capable of symptom relief. The development of levodopa in the 1960s took over nine years of research and trials, with the first clinical trials showing negative or, at best, uncertain benefits. However, once levodopa was approved and released, its almost legendary prowess at relieving a wide range of PD symptoms set a rather high bar for other drugs to meet. Amantadine, the next medication to be developed, was recognized as having extra benefits for relieving tremors that were not achieved by all patients receiving levodopa. Thereafter, clinical trials began to take on therapeutic goals that targeted deficiencies in levodopa treatments.

By participating in a clinical trial, patients have the opportunity to test out the latest advances in medications. Though there is always some risk in testing a newly developed drug (the risks include potential side effects or unforeseen rare adverse reactions), there are always safety constraints imposed upon the trialed drugs by the FDA and a local institutional review board (IRB). Some patients would prefer just to receive the active drug rather than the study placebo, which is an inevitable concomitant of all modern pharmaceutical research. Of course, if a drug in a study were to be found to have an unanticipated toxicity, one might prefer to have been on the "sugar pill" rather than the active drug.

Current clinical trials are testing therapies that attempt to improve upon current levodopa products by increasing potency and extending the duration of efficacy (like the dopaminergic agonists discussed earlier in this chapter). Drugs that can block involuntary movements and hallucinations have been developed through clinical research in efforts to tone down unwanted actions of levodopa. The most recent drug released for adjunctive use in advanced PD, istradefylline, was approved by the FDA more than 10 years after its last US clinical trial was completed. This drug is used for lessening "off" time, meaning the experience of being undermedicated. As illustrated by the experience with istradefylline, the testing process and FDA approval can take years before a drug can be released for prescription purposes.

No matter where you are on your PD journey, but especially if you are newly diagnosed, you should work closely with your care team to determine which medication or combination of medications is best for you and your symptoms. Often it is a process of trial and error that results in the best dose of a medication or the combination of two or more. Keep in mind that the information presented in this book, particularly surrounding medications, should be used only for reference and never be construed as a prescription for a particular medication or treatment regimen. Always consult with your physician at the onset of your symptoms and for the duration in order to maintain the best course of treatment.

Surgical Intervention

As we've seen, loss of nerve cells is the hallmark of brain changes in PD. The consequences of these neurodegenerative changes are alterations in the functioning of brain circuits between one group of nerve cells and another group. Since there is considerable scientific proof demonstrating how these pathways function, the next step was for laboratory scientists to develop ideas for performing surgery on the brain with hopes of modulating these circuits for therapeutic purposes. Clinical experimental trials starting in the 1980s proved that there were reasons to use invasive procedures in order to alter these pathways. So, although medications are the primary course of therapeutics for most patients, surgical procedures within the brain have become an established option for those with advanced PD. Most people with newly diagnosed PD will never need these neurosurgical treatments, and so the following discussion is in the interest of education rather than planning for the inevitable.

DEEP BRAIN STIMULATION

Beginning in the 1990s, neurosurgical researchers started to investigate the therapeutic potential of implanted electronic stimulatory devices in the brain that functioned in ways like heart pacemakers. The devices contained small, powerful batteries capable of stimulating, or sending out electrical pulses that would continuously alleviate the symptoms of PD for years. These devices, called implantable pulse generators, were adjustable in terms of their output voltage, pulse frequency, and other settings useful for optimizing the effects. These devices and the electrodes (wires placed within the brain and connected to the electrical pulse generators) form the basis of a therapy called deep brain stimulation (DBS). The "deep brain" wording in this term refers to the fact that the electrode is implanted several inches deep in the brain, since the appropriate targets for electrical stimulation require such localization. Today, DBS is widely used internationally and in a manner that hasn't changed much in many years. It is generally chosen for specific PD problems that have been unresponsive to medications; in other words, it's not a treatment for patients newly diagnosed with PD. The only instance in which DBS might be used for a newly diagnosed PD patient would be for that extremely rare situation in which a bothersome tremor would be inadequately controlled by trials of all available medications.

Today, DBS has come a long way from being experimental, and it is not regarded as a high-risk procedure. Enough research has been done and knowledge gained about DBS to understand what it can and cannot improve. Patients with imbalance or swallowing problems, for example, do not benefit from DBS. A few patients with freezing of gait have seen benefit from DBS, but most do not, so most DBS centers would not recommend performing DBS for freezing of gait even if it's not effectively controlled by medication. DBS also does not slow the progression of PD or prevent the eventual development of motor impairments.

In recent years, research has been done on earlier uses of DBS. In these studies, patients not meeting criteria for conventional use of DBS—intractable tremor, dyskinesias (uncontrolled, involuntary muscle movements caused by levodopa therapy), "off" time (repeated episodes of suboptimal medication benefits) not well controlled with all available drug options—were given DBS and studied for several years. The results indicated that the incidence of dyskinesias and motor fluctuations was lower than in those who had not been treated with DBS. These findings suggested that DBS alleviated or prevented these problems. However, the interpretation of these results is confounded by the fact that the treatment tested for avoidance of the problems is the same treatment that would mask the future arrival of such symptoms. Presently, newly diagnosed patients are not candidates for DBS, because medications can work so well. DBS is FDA-approved for use earlier than the five-year or greater time point at which it is currently used in most treatment centers in the United States.

THALAMOTOMY AND PALLIDOTOMY

Thalamotomy (a small surgically placed burn, or lesion, in a portion of the brain called the thalamus) and pallidotomy (a surgical lesion in the brain's structure called the globus pallidus interna, abbreviated as GPi) are procedures that were used several decades ago for treating PD, but today they are rarely, if ever, employed. As mentioned on page 59 with respect to DBS, an intervention that alters specific portions of brain circuitry can improve upon the effects of PD medications. This finding became known to physicians after studying the effects of strokes on just those brain regions that are now targeted for improving PD symptoms; the outcomes from such strokes included immediate improvement of tremors and other Parkinsonian features. Based on these rare experiences, researchers reasoned that intentionally interrupting specific pathways in the brain that control motor functions could lead to improvements in a safe and reliable manner.

The benefits of surgical intervention for PD were first demonstrated with thalamotomy, carried out in the 1960s to relieve PD tremors. Thalamotomy is carried out by a neurosurgeon, who carefully identifies a specific minute portion of the thalamus called the ventral intermediate (VIM) nucleus. This location is very specific for relief of tremors, and the selective damage placed there lacks any other neurological consequences. By interrupting brain signals passing through the VIM nucleus, tremors can be relieved permanently. Of course, medications offer a much simpler and safer way to achieve the goal of tremor relief, especially since VIM thalamotomy is not without its risks. Today, DBS targeting the VIM nucleus in the thalamus is the treatment of choice rather than thalamotomy. Clinical experience has shown that thalamotomy should be restricted to treating just one side of the brain, because of the risk in some patients for causing speech and swallowing problems if this treatment is carried out on both sides of the brain. In contrast, DBS targeted at the thalamus on both sides of the brain for improving bilateral tremor can be carried out safely.

Newer Techniques for Treating PD

Both pallidotomy and thalamotomy (see definitions on page 60) are only rarely carried out today because of the widespread use of DBS. The electrical stimulation settings in DBS can be adjusted in the outpatient clinic to improve symptom control and to avoid possible side effects. In contrast, pallidotomy and thalamotomy lead to permanent lesions in the brain. If the proper target has been missed or the lesion is an incorrect size, the lesioning procedures (thalamotomy or pallidotomy) may fail to achieve the desired results. For more than 20 years, DBS has replaced brain lesioning for PD. This situation might change in the future, however, based on a new methodology called focused ultrasound (FUS). FUS is a nonsurgical way to achieve the same outcomes previously offered by pallidotomy and thalamotomy. The full name of this new procedure is magnetic resonance–guided focused ultrasound (MRG-FUS). The idea behind MRG-FUS is that energy via ultrasound waves can be beamed quite selectively at the VIM thalamus nucleus or the GPi in order to accomplish circuitry interruptions that previously required a brain operation and insertion of a heated electrode. No surgery is needed for MRG-FUS. Instead, this technique involves placing a patient in a conventional MRI scanner. Surrounding the head are devices that beam into the skull narrow beams of high-power ultrasound waves. A short burst of ultrasound waves is beamed into a location carefully determined by MRI. The beams within the MRI unit come from multiple directions, and only where they intersect is a thalamotomy or pallidotomy carried out. Ultrasound waves can then be beamed toward the proper region of the brain in order to eradicate tremors. MRG-FUS is currently approved in the United States for treating tremor. FUS of the GPi for achieving pallidotomy has been tried experimentally but isn't approved in the United States. Whether these newer techniques will ultimately be judged to be the equal of DBS or will differ in options for patients remains to be learned. Currently, MRG-FUS is also approved only for one side of the brain (just like pallidotomy and thalamotomy); it is possible that this limitation might also change in the future.

For the newly diagnosed PD patient with tremor, MRG-FUS is not likely to be used as an initial treatment. Only if tremor is not adequately controlled would this be considered. There hasn't been extensive long-term experience with FUS, and there are possibly some risks that haven't been determined to date. As mentioned on page 53, most patients respond so well to conventional medications for tremor that there won't be the need for undergoing any additional treatment, invasive or non-invasive, beyond dopaminergic therapy.

As we've seen, there are a wide range of available therapeutic options to treat PD. They can be as simple as a few levodopa pills taken daily. To get the best results from this and the other types of PD medications, it is important to maintain communication with your prescriber so that medication decisions can be helped by experienced guidance. The team approach to the management of PD offers support from several disciplines and specialties, and it's good to take advantage of all available professional opinions (such as those of your physician and pharmacist). Currently, there are active research studies happening with the goal of devising new treatments for PD, both medications and surgical procedures.

In the next chapter, we'll cover another very important component in managing your PD: your family members and caretakers. It's your disorder and ultimately up to you how you navigate it, but those around you want to help. We'll discuss the best ways for communicating your diagnosis to others and where you can turn for help in facing the daily challenges of living with PD.

CHAPTER 4
Family Members
and Caretakers

Having PD can make one feel alone, and the "why me" feelings may give way to a deeply felt conclusion that an isolated existence with this disorder is inevitable. Many patients experience a sense of separation from those around them, based on several reasons. For one, the outward appearance of PD on the face and the rest of the body can be a caricature of advanced aging and frailty. Even with the mildest of symptoms and a picture of PD that is barely diagnosable by a physician meeting you for the first time, the new identity of having PD can be loaded with socially stigmatizing problems. Let's start with the impact of tremor, as seen by others. The shaking hands of PD can be misinterpreted in many ways, sometimes inaccurately. Since tremors increase in any stressful situation (pleasant or otherwise), well-meaning family and friends may read into the tremor other ongoing problems for you, such as anxiety, weakness, and, worst of all, misuse of alcohol or drugs. Because tremor is so apparent to others, trying to disguise it carries the risk of being perceived as attempting to hide a more ominous disorder. Patients should consider that those in the circle around them probably have discerned their tremor from time to time. If so, they might be reacting to it with some degree of worry, perhaps even misperception of the tremor as signaling a dire health problem. An employer's view of tremors could be such that a PD patient's continued work might be in jeopardy because of future incapacity in a variety of work settings. And children, who sometimes say the darndest things, can also be a challenge for explaining what it's all about in simplified concepts that they can understand.

I sometimes find that the most successful adaptations to living with PD have to do with a patient's close circle—a spouse, children, even close friends—taking on the identity of "we." We have PD, we are changing the medication schedule, we are getting out to the exercise class. PD is not a hereditary or contagious disorder, but taking outward measures to counteract the sense of isolation can, in my opinion, make therapeutic inroads into this disorder. This notion of PD fosters a sense of teamwork. Motivation for improving endurance in exercise, for trying to increase socialization, and for fighting back against personal stereotypes of what it is to be "ill" is best found in company. PD is unique among neurological disorders and health problems in general because it allows patients this choice of creating a shared goal with others.

At the same time you are assembling your support team, you can be quite explicit in the rules they need to observe with you. Especially with mild PD, the door doesn't need to be held open for you, and your possessions don't have to be carried by others. If you have a soft voice or slowed speech, others do not need to finish your sentences. People who are hard of hearing may give you signals from time to time about speaking louder, however. Since this is such a common problem, and since a diminished volume of your voice might not be perceived by you, learning to take this feedback gracefully may be one of the concessions you may have to make. After all, those around you want to hear from you everything said. The message I'm trying to convey is that your care team may have very few roles to fulfill in enhancing your comfort, safety, and functioning in everyday life. One patient I recall was especially annoyed by the fact that others always seemed to be wanting to make her a passenger when going out for a drive, with the implicit assumption that driving was more difficult (or less safe) because of her PD diagnosis. Advanced forms of PD can affect the ability to drive (see page 85), but not all people with PD have this difficulty. A clear statement of the details of one's abilities and disabilities should be a topic of discussion in establishing caregiver relationships.

A final comment: This book, like anything written about PD, necessarily has to generalize and stereotype. As important as it might be for having a supportive community of friends and family, wouldn't it be nice if PD wasn't even on everyone's radar? Sometimes people with PD do have such a good level of symptom control that it doesn't have to be a topic of observation by others or an identity change. "Disguised PD" is a term I have heard from some persons who have a strong opinion that denial of the diagnosis (at least as far as others are concerned) seems to be the way they wish to lead their life. Since outcomes of PD can often be quite benign, I sometimes endorse this attitude in discussion with patients. I also try to give honest feedback as to whether others might discern some inkling of the presence of PD or something that might elicit concern by others. Given the effectiveness of medications to mask outward features of PD, some persons with the diagnosis of PD may have the luxury of going about their lives unhindered by the PD identity.

Breaking the News

When the news of a PD diagnosis is shared with your family, friends, coworkers, and others you choose to know, how should this be worded? If you have hand tremors, keep in mind that these likely have been observed by others. Some might correctly have anticipated this admission by you. Others might have suspected another disorder with tremor, including the possibility that the neurological condition was essential tremor, a disorder much more common in the general population and characterized by a tremor arising only during activity of the hands. Keep in mind that once medication has been started, most or all of your symptoms might vanish to those around you, never to reemerge if you are fortunate. However, there is a good chance that some outward inkling of Parkinsonism might be evident to those familiar with you. So, disguising your diagnosis might not be the best strategy for living with PD. It may be useful to develop a simple script that provides you with a straightforward explanation. One version of talking points might be something like this: "You may be wondering where that tremor comes from. Well, I'm told by a neurologist that it's Parkinson's, though I'm calling it just a nuisance at the moment. I'm getting it treated, and I feel like I'm back to normal." A brief statement like that has been used by a few people I've known. It can serve the purpose of dispelling worry in listeners, especially since this type of message conveys that you have availed yourself of a competent evaluation and treatment.

Given the age at which PD often intrudes in your life, it's not uncommon that relatively young children, such as grandchildren, may need to get to know this malady. Older children also have the ability to orient themselves in their relationship with you around a sound footing in what PD is and isn't. Here's some commonsense advice on how to envision the sharing of information about your diagnosis: Don't keep it hidden. A tremoring hand stuffed in a pocket may provide temporary or insufficient disguise. The child perceiving something is "wrong" with you may imagine far worse problems, including fear about your longevity or suffering. Since they are related to you, you can explain that it's not (except very rarely) an inherited condition, and it certainly isn't caused by being in the presence of someone with PD. It might be best not to assume that these facts will be known to a child. Maybe you shouldn't be the only source of information; you can suggest another family member amplify what you have shared. You might envision spreading your story of living with PD by planning to speak about it on another occasion to emphasize that discussion of PD is not off-limits as far as you are concerned.

Fortunately, there are many books for children on the topic of PD. Some of the best introductions to the topic are a series of books available from a British PD advocacy group, Parkinsons UK (Parkinsons.org.uk). These five short volumes are nicely illustrated, clearly written, and available free of charge by download from this organization's website. There are many other books out there with similar themes. Children heading toward middle-school age might also be motivated to write reports about PD as classwork, and so your malady may become a topic of expertise that you can share with the younger generation as they get to know what you experience with PD.

Creating empathy with someone affected by PD—ah, there's the challenge! Especially for someone newly diagnosed or fortunate to have continued in good control of symptoms, sympathy may be unwelcome. Establishing and continuing with an empathetic relationship will likely require a careful interpretation of even the style of communication. For example, most persons are not "suffering" with PD, nor are they necessarily disabled. The friends and family may be as uncertain of what's ahead as the PD patient (and the treating physician as well), but assuming progression to a pitiable state needs to be avoided by others. This can be accomplished by good communication with the circle of family and friends. There is enough information for a lay audience about what PD is—and isn't—that the myths can be dispelled. A reduced life span, the need for moving to a safer home, and a higher risk of falls and choking, for example, are erroneous perceptions that have arisen among concerned family and caregivers for people whose current experience with PD includes none of these issues. Perhaps the most important lesson that friends and family should learn alongside the PD patient is to develop a heightened sense of optimism about living with PD, now and in the future. The odds support such optimism, and self-education, asking questions of authoritative sources, and recognizing that everyone with PD has a highly individualized experience can lead to the best outcome in avoiding isolation for the PD patient.

Maintaining Your Autonomy

Are you now in control of your destiny? A bit philosophical, I realize, but if we sum up life with PD, do you still feel in control of decisions about yourself in the context of your family, your working environment, and so on? Just because you have PD doesn't mean you have to plan for a new home, premature retirement, and dependency, but others may think so. At the same time, when you may be somewhat in the dark as to what's ahead, the world around you might have a much more dire, and inappropriate, view of living with PD. You may be placed in the new role of defending the relatively benign experience of PD against misperceptions. It might be necessary to get the input of your neurologist or some other authoritative source to back up your assertion of autonomy for the way you feel decisions should be made. It's not an inappropriate request for you to make of your treating physician. Be gentle with the sincere feelings of your caregivers, especially if they mean well and are lacking in good information about your PD experience. Your personal boundaries need to be respected. For example, no one disputes that exercise is good for you and that we all need encouragement from time to time. However, a spouse who passionately argues for a daily hour-long workout at the gym in the hopes of slowing PD may be promoting too much of a good idea that can become burdensome (unless you're enjoying all that exercise!).

Navigating Changing Relationships

Any new interaction with physicians and any new diagnosis carry the risk of what medical sociologists have called the "sick role," meaning that decisions and perceptions of daily life may be colored or even overwhelmed by a diagnosis like PD. This does not mean that someone new to PD is likely to become a hypochondriac, a constant complainer, or sunk in despair. The fact that PD is, at present, an incurable disorder may resonate more deeply for some persons than for others. In some instances, no rationalization based on comparison with other illnesses like cancer and heart disease (both of which threaten survival, after all) provides comfort to those who may have taken on the "sick role." It becomes the task of someone newly diagnosed with PD and at intervals thereafter to adopt a personal philosophy of quality living. Much of this philosophy will be guided by crafting strong relationships with others. A phrase I remember from listening to a patient describe an upcoming Caribbean cruise, "in spite of PD, I . . .," signifies the kind of relationship achieved with the inner self and with others that can be the goal of navigating the future.

Generally, PD intrudes in your life at an age when other indignities of the decades you have lived are also making themselves known. Stiff and sometimes painful joints, fragmented sleep from bathroom trips, and a medication cabinet with too many pills can crowd out the unique role that PD might have in your life. You may be seeing your neurologist for matters other than PD, such as neuropathy (a loss of full feeling in the longest nerves of your body in the feet, a common aging-related problem) or lower-back pains.

You may start to encounter other physicians who might know less about PD than you do. A situation I've heard repeatedly has been worry on the part of an orthopedic surgeon that recovery after a knee or hip replacement operation will be problematic for everyone with PD (it won't be, of course). Relationships with other physicians may also lead you to discover that many of them are not all that well informed about PD. The growing list of PD medications may be unfamiliar, for example. Patients who lack a tremor may be puzzling to a primary care physician who might suspect that shaking is a mandatory feature of a correct diagnosis. My advice is not to lose faith in your medical specialist just because he or she may seem to know less than you, a PD patient who has researched the topic. One of your new roles in the postdiagnosis world is to serve as a new source of education to the medical community by sharing your personal experience with PD.

Another challenging set of relationships has to do with people in the wider world beyond established family connections and old friends. The digital age has created opportunities at your fingertips (or through voice-activated dictation in most modern home computers) for communicating with anyone in the world with virtually no cost other than your time. Many patients have learned to find others with PD through chat groups, blogs, and other social media connections. Facebook and other Internet platforms abound in PD-related sites. Those living far away from the locations of support groups can join so-called virtual support groups throughout the United States and elsewhere. Questions that can be answered by linking with others through social media can range from getting the best price on medications to the best walkers for balance support or the latest information on new clinical trials. Certain portions of the PD demographic—those with young age of onset, for example—are often especially interested in online relationships with others similarly affected. Online friendships that develop also offer the opportunity to get to know someone without needing to mention one's health background, like the diagnosis of PD. Even if PD handwriting would make a written letter difficult to read, the advent of electronic text has become the great equalizer!

When Additional Help Is Needed

Living well with PD can be achieved as a solitary experience. That said, there are many situations when the help of others can greatly improve quality of life. Let me provide a few examples:

A common concern for persons with PD, especially those over the age of 70, is whether driving an automobile is safe or not. (This topic is discussed in further detail on page 85.) For those who wish to continue driving (and thereby maintain an important part of their autonomy), there can be an apparent impasse with family members who have their own strong feelings on the topic. Their concerns may be well founded, of course. There can also be too much willingness by family members to permit driving by someone whose skills behind the wheel are suspect. For both situations, additional help is needed by an impartial individual who is willing to drive with the PD person and make an objective judgment as to safety. This can be done in an empty parking lot, if necessary. This assessment should be followed by a written version. In some communities, there are resources for formal assessment by occupational therapists, sometimes equipped with driving simulators or similar options. This professional assessment may be expensive. The state motor vehicle department also can provide a road test.

Independence is an unspoken goal for just about everyone with PD at all stages of the disorder. If problems with mobility, balance, or self-care arise, as they will for some after a few years, the helping hands of others may become necessary. These tasks often start off small, like placing arms in sleeves, but then transition to tasks that are more physically demanding. Healthy spouses or other household caregivers may welcome these roles and find them not to be an imposition. However, tasks involving lifting and bending or disrupted sleep can easily overburden a life companion. The transition to such demands can be gradual. When help is needed, there might not be many options that are easily affordable. Home care aides are available in many communities from agencies that have bonded workers and some flexibility in when they can come to the home. Often there is a required three- to four-hour service minimum. Generally, they do not provide out-of-home transportation or home cleaning as part of the services provided. Supervision against falls, bathing, preparation of meals, and companionship are provided, often at a price that is acceptable (and possibly covered by supplemental long-term care insurance). The Veterans Administration (VA) is one potential source of support.

CHAPTER 5
Living with Parkinson's

A diagnosis of PD often means that lifestyle changes are ahead, including modifying or renovating your home (or even purchasing a new home), special employment arrangements for people who are still working, and increased reliance on family members, friends, and caretakers, as discussed in chapter 4. You may also find that the way you relate to your partner or spouse may change. In this chapter, we'll explore some of the practical challenges of living with PD and offer useful tips on how you can take charge and be proactive in these important areas of your life.

Support Groups

Since the 1960s, support groups for PD have flourished around the world. In the United States, assemblies of PD patients and their caregivers are common in many communities. Sometimes a local or statewide organization takes on a coordination role, often enlisting local professional assistance from physicians, nurses, or other health care personnel to offer advisory structure and authoritative advice to these group meetings. Some support groups take "all comers," while others try to specialize in content aimed at particular members of the PD community, such as those with young-onset PD or those still employed who seek workplace advice. Caregivers, especially those dealing with more advanced PD patients or PD patients who have additional physical or mental disabilities, may also find support and useful information in their own assemblies, separately from those for whom they provide care.

Should you join a support group? Consider these questions when making a decision: Do you like the idea of being among like-minded individuals with PD (and their caregivers)? Does the idea of seeing many other PD patients whose symptoms may be lighter or much worse than yours bother you? Will it be depressing to see the full range of the impacts of PD? Will you be able to take away something positive from being around other people with PD? And in turn, can you contribute something positive to a support group that might give a sense of purpose to a person coping with PD? These and other questions are worth pondering if you're interested in attending a support group.

Fortunately, these questions are easily answered by the experience of actually attending a support group. It might not be a familiar experience for you to bond with others through a particular malady, and it might be uncomfortable or overwhelming at first to see many others with various outward expressions of PD, but this is one of the best things you can do for your mental health: surround yourself with others who share the same affliction as you. You may be surprised by how much support and camaraderie you can glean just by being around others with PD, speaking with them, and hearing their stories. Many people who meet in support groups become lifelong friends, and often other elements of support flow from this affiliation, such as shared transportation, tips on treatments and coping mechanisms, and engaging in joint exercise classes. Of course, there is the possibility that you may not get anything useful or beneficial from attending a support group, and this is okay, too—there is never an obligation to keep attending. In urban areas where there may be several group meetings, you will likely have more options among which to choose the best mix of program content, attendees, and scheduling. Some groups offer specific themes such as young-onset PD, exercise or dance programs, guest health care professionals to offer tips and advice, or monthly educational speakers. Many national and regional organizations ensure that the leaders of their support groups have a strong background or are highly educated in the disorder and are able to lead and moderate the meetings effectively. For many individuals whose experience with PD has left them feeling overwhelmed or even stigmatized by their social contacts, a regular support group meeting becomes their ticket back into the world of others. If you're someone who is handling their PD well, you might consider participating in a support group to lend support and optimism to those who may be having a more difficult time navigating their own experience with the disorder.

Helpful Tools and Gadgets

Over the years, I've heard from PD patients about many items they use to help make their lives easier. Among these items, the electric toothbrush stands out from the rest. It can become a much-appreciated aid on a daily basis, because the repetitive movements required for good brushing are often impaired, even in those with mild PD. In selecting which brand and model to choose, I can't advise, because they are all similar in my mind (and most have equal or comparable functions). But if you share the toothbrush handle with others, pay attention to the ease of attaching and detaching the brush head when you switch out the brush head, because the dexterity involved may be the important differentiator.

Since tremors and decreased dexterity are common symptoms even with mild PD, another nuisance has to do with buttoning clothing. Especially for dress shirts, the tiny buttons involved can mean torment for dressing and undressing. Fortunately, there are ways to get around buttons. Having small segments of Velcro installed at the sites of button closures can resolve the problem with no need to purchase a new wardrobe. There is also a buttoning aid that loops around buttons so that they can be tugged into place; without too much searching, these can easily be found on the Internet. Other items that can help in the tasks of dressing include a long-handled shoehorn, sock extenders to pull socks onto feet, and short sticks (or that shoehorn) that can aid putting arms in sleeves.

For those who find that, because of PD, keyboard typing has become slowed or imprecise, this may be the time to take advantage of dictation software. As you speak through a small headset microphone or the microphone on your computer, your words will appear on the screen instantly. This dictation can be used for emails, blogs, recipes, letters, reminders, or the start of your Great American Novel.

You might find an enlarged computer keyboard to be helpful for improving the precision of typing. Models with raised keys almost double the size of conventional keyboards are widely available on the Internet. One source is Adaptive Tech Solutions (AdaptiveTechSolutions.com), which has a keyboard with Bluetooth so that extra cords aren't needed. Use of a rollerball mouse can be easier than the conventional mouse, especially if tremor makes it difficult to target the mouse. Two other items that can be useful (also available from Adaptive Tech Solutions) are a portable voice amplifier and an adjustable gooseneck stand that can grasp and position a tablet for easy viewing.

Of course, there are many other items on the market that can offer improved convenience. Many of these items can be found in catalogs or websites that are targeted to seniors or those living with disabilities such as PD. One example is a vegetable chopper, which allows you to prepare meals without the use of sharp knives. Another is a set of satin fabric sheets that, together with silk or satin pajamas, can make navigation in bed much less of an effort. Look for a set that has flannel or cotton edges; this addition avoids the risk of sliding around too much in bed.

In addition to the mental and emotional support offered by support groups, they are also often sources of useful information that you may not find elsewhere. Recommendations for caring and competent physicians, prices on medication, exercise classes, and local PD research opportunities, like clinical trials, can be shared in these groups. Meetings can also be a place where myths are dispelled, jokes or stories are shared, and practical guidance can be given as to how to explain this disorder to others. Not all support group meetings succeed on all counts, but the chances are good for getting useful information and more when you attend a support group. Most support groups are governed democratically, meaning that the leaders will look to the members for what type of content and activities they'd like to learn or engage in. No matter where you are on your PD journey, seeking out and building a community with others who are affected by the disease can be essential. Finding like-minded people, both patients and caregivers, with whom you can share experiences and information is an important component in taking charge of this disorder.

Getting Around

It isn't just futurists who tell us that self-driving cars are soon to be part of our lives; the automobile industry is already producing such vehicles. Nevertheless, since those cars are not the mainstream yet, humans are still responsible for operating vehicles, which means they must be able to do so safely and responsibly. Driving is one of the major everyday functions that can be significantly affected by PD. In the early stages of the disease, a person may be able to continue driving perfectly well without any interference from their symptoms or medications. However, as the disease progresses, driving can become increasingly dangerous both for the person driving with PD and for others on the road. PD poses a special challenge, because the driver who acquires PD generally does not want to give up the privilege of driving and the freedom it allows. For someone who has a long driving career characterized by prior safe performance, giving up driving can be difficult, but it is something that must be seriously considered by the patient and their caregiver. Some people with PD clearly should not be driving, particularly if they have limited vision or limited ability to turn their neck from side to side to look around them, or if tremors make it difficult to maintain control over the wheel or the gas and brake pedals. Sometimes the reason that someone with PD shouldn't drive is because of factors other than PD itself. As we know, PD often intersects with advanced age, where the question of limited or no driving is raised as a matter of course due to limited mobility, decreased vision, and other age-related symptoms. When the question is raised as to whether or not it's safe for a person with PD to continue driving, they should be evaluated by an objective person they trust, whether it's a neighbor or a care provider who can assess their driving skills. Perhaps one of the best ways to make this assessment is to take a drive in an empty parking lot with an observer taking note of capabilities with brakes and the steering wheel. If the person is observed to be driving dangerously, such as wandering across pavement lines, not using proper signals, not applying the brakes safely, or generally being unsafe behind the wheel, taking away the keys from them must be seriously considered in order to protect them and other drivers, bicyclists, and pedestrians.

The Critical Role of Self-Compassion

How do you step outside of the burden of living with PD? Do you seek out a way to contemplate the good things in your life with as much attention and appreciation as you would like to balance out the stumbles and shakes of PD? A first step in this direction is to assess your mental health by analyzing whether there are elements of depression or anxiety in your everyday experience. You might ask those around you for guidance on this as well. If so, keep in mind that it is no sign of weakness to seek out help from a medical practitioner or psychologist. You might be relieved to learn that you're not alone in these experiences, and there are available treatments and people to listen and help.

Another way to coax compassion out of your deepest feelings about yourself is through a discipline called *mindfulness*. Mindfulness is a contemplative means for stress reduction that you can easily add to your day's activities. This special time offers relaxation and a mind-focusing experience that might be explored in the context of yoga exercises, sitting amid favorite aromas, concentrating on breathing exercises, flower arranging, or a host of other activities. Sometimes it can be a group activity, as with Tai Chi or yoga classes; for others, it's a private time when you examine your habits, your positivity, your unwelcome and excessive expectations of yourself, and so on. There's a lot of reading available on this topic. With respect to PD, there has been an investigation of mindfulness as a means to achieve improved functioning. This topic is reviewed in a 2015 online-accessible article by PD specialist Barbara Pickut, MD, published in the journal *Parkinson's Disease*. Dr. Pickut and colleagues found that a specific course of mindfulness behavioral intervention in 27 PD patients led to a reduction in PD symptoms as well as other improvements. A daily habit of putting aside time for a mindfulness exercise may pay off in ways that you might not have expected.

Mindfulness can also take the form of regularly working toward a physical achievement goal that might seem outside the realm of the stereotype of PD. For example, contemplating that some of my elderly patients (men and women) would be engaging regularly in boxing certainly raised my eyebrows a few years ago, but no longer. In my community and throughout the world, thousands of people are gaining exercise and self-confidence through this well-structured activity (see RockSteadyBoxing.org for further information and its magazine). Other forms of exercise are especially conducive to the PD cause. For example, for those whose balance is impaired, there's nothing like warm-water pool exercise wearing a float belt, as it provides all the exercise you need for your legs and lower back with no risk of falls. And don't overlook throwing darts for enhancing your concentration. One of my patients with the worst resting tremor found that his aim was true when he threw darts, and he regularly won bets from those who doubted his skill!

Should you be driving if you have PD? Among the ways to approach this question can be an honest self-appraisal of whether near-accidents or other unsafe situations have occurred. If driving seems to bring out anxiety or unsafe performance behind the wheel, this might be a clue that driving should be a thing of the past. A symptom of PD can be slowed reaction times, which could influence braking or sudden turns. It should be said that receiving a diagnosis of PD does not require the motor vehicle department or one's car insurance agent to be notified. Medications for PD (particularly dopaminergic agonists) can be sedating, but there is no obligation to limit driving because of medications unless daytime drowsiness is a problem. Sometimes the biggest challenge with driving is not being on the road but finding a close parking spot if walking poses difficulties. PD patients are entitled to handicap parking placards, and they shouldn't be afraid to obtain one if they feel that walking ability is compromised.

Finally, the decision as to whether or not to continue driving might be tempered by consideration of the alternatives. Since one's driving ability might change for the worse in the future, perhaps the present is ideal for reconsidering the need to maintain a personal automobile, especially if its use is becoming less frequent or necessary (if you're no longer working, for example). One might also weigh the cost of automobile ownership against the cost of using local taxis, rideshare apps, or public transportation. And for those living in areas where the weather is relatively mild year-round, bicycles can be rediscovered as a useful and fun way of getting around. (Many communities offer bicycles that can be rented by the hour and have convenient pickup and drop-off locations.) Even though balance can be impaired when walking, the PD patient on a bicycle often has excellent balance (since the stability of bicycles is generated by the gyroscope effect of the wheels).

Setting Up Your Home

With a diagnosis of PD, it's prudent to start thinking about modifications to your home for improved accessibility. Similar considerations are generally thought about when simply getting older, to account for the possibility of diminished mobility regardless of the specific symptoms PD might cause, but keep in mind that most persons with PD are generally not disabled to the extent that major home renovations are necessary, even at five years or more after diagnosis. Remember that progression of PD looks different for everyone, and that a milestone of about three years postdiagnosis often provides guidance as to what your lifetime experience with PD might look like. If you are in a position to make certain choices that require financial consideration, you might think about the possibility of living in a one-story home, given the uncertainties ahead and the potential decrease in mobility (which again, often happens naturally with age, regardless of PD). If you have plans for renovations to kitchens or bathrooms, you might take into consideration some modifications for increased safety, such as grab bars on countertops or in doorways. Both kitchens and bathrooms are high on the list of most common sites for at-home falls among older individuals and individuals with disabilities. Despite these considerations, also keep in mind that for many patients with longstanding PD, even those with known balance problems, stairways with sturdy banisters may be perfectly safe to navigate. The more pertinent risk for falling for patients with PD can be walking in settings where they're likely to back up or make turns (such as in closets or hallways).

Some reasonable adaptations should be considered to lessen risks for falls. Sturdy grab bars should be placed in showers, bathtubs, and near the toilet in bathrooms. Medicare may support the cost of these items. An expert review of your home can be performed by the nonprofit Visiting Nurse Association or another home health care agency. Such services can advise on detailed measures to improve safety, such as the removal of loose towel bars and upgrades of toilet seats with handles on the side.

The purpose of all these modifications is simply to make living with PD easier and more enjoyable. Of course, they may not apply to every person with PD, but you can take the suggestions that are helpful and tailor them to your own situation. Whatever is within your means to accomplish, even small changes (such as installing grab bars in your bathroom and kitchen) will make everyday living easier.

Navigating the Workplace

For people living with PD who continue to work outside of the home, many questions may arise, sometimes right after diagnosis. One fear that I have heard multiple times from patients is that they will immediately be deemed unfit for work and therefore will be unable to maintain a livelihood. An opposing viewpoint a patient might take, which also depends on age and financial situation, is that it's time to retire and get some enjoyment out of life while they're still in relatively good health. Neither of these views fully captures the complete picture of living with PD, but each is valid in reflecting how all of us think from time to time. I won't attempt to generalize about all types of employment in this section, but I can state with confidence that leaving the workforce is only rarely necessary due to the onset of PD. Specialized situations may sometimes necessitate this, for example, in the case of a commercial airline pilot (and in this situation, because of using certain medications for PD, not the diagnosis alone). A performer whose voice suffers from PD will of course have a problem continuing their work, but the majority of PD patients maintain effective speech even if symptoms, such as a reduction in loudness or clarity, develop after several years. The greatest challenges concerning those with PD in the workplace have to do with perceptions (especially misperceptions) by employers. Often with an unrealistic view of PD, an employer or the human resources department may jump to a conclusion that disability is inevitable and that the employee's job performance will suffer or decline. There may also be the erroneous concern that medical expenses for that person will soar, especially if there is in-house concern about a self-funded medical coverage plan. In businesses dependent on sales or other types of negotiations, an employer may envision a PD patient becoming less effective or not presenting well on behalf of the company. Jobs with physical demands might be perceived as likely to become too difficult or unsafe to accomplish. And then there are the patient's own concerns, which can include fears of being fired or becoming unable to keep up with the pace or demands of their work.

The advice I can offer includes waiting until symptomatic medication has been effectively managed to achieve optimal treatment of PD signs and symptoms before any decisions

Parkinson's and Pregnancy

Rarely, PD can develop during a woman's reproductive years. The good news is that PD is not known to interfere with fertility or the nine-month course of pregnancy. Many healthy babies have been born to women with PD. Most physicians would not discourage such a pregnancy, although there may be some increased challenges along the way. For example, if medications are needed for control of symptoms, none of them are classified as being appropriate for use during pregnancy. A mother-to-be should consider the possibilities of getting through the nine months in the absence of symptomatic treatment, if possible. If not, there is considerable reported evidence that levodopa-carbidopa use has not led to congenital malformations and fetal development problems. Nevertheless, medication use cannot be recommended during pregnancy, especially during the first trimester. Another challenge is posed by the exacerbation of PD symptoms, such as increased tremors, that can arise as a physiological consequence of pregnancy. This isn't a major effect in most instances. Interested parties can review several reports in the medical literature on this topic. PD doesn't seem to cause difficulties in labor and delivery. Nursing a baby is not affected, though if symptomatic medication for PD needs to be taken in the postpartum period, keep in mind that the drugs can be transported via breast milk to the baby. Most important, though PD does present unique physical and emotional challenges, it should not be a reason for a woman not to pursue pregnancy and motherhood if that is what she wishes.

are made. Often this might require several weeks, as some drugs might need to be tried and adjusted over such a period of time. Although accommodations might not be necessary in the workplace, some activities might be unsuitable even for a typical patient with relatively mild PD (activities such as climbing ladders or work tasks requiring a great deal of keyboarding or handwriting).

HOW AND WHEN TO DISCLOSE

On the topic of informing your employer about your PD, you may wonder whether that is even a good idea. Your personal medical history is, of course, a private matter, and you have no obligation to share it with anyone, especially someone who could conceivably use this information against you. But keep in mind that should you opt not to disclose your condition, it may lead to other undesirable outcomes. The resting tremor of someone with PD can easily be misinterpreted as something else that poses an obvious risk to employment, such as alcoholism or illicit drug use. Someone with tremors might be perceived as especially anxious or insecure in their job. Other aspects of PD can also be regarded by others with alarm and suspicion. Again, whether and how you disclose your diagnosis is up to you, but it might be strategic to let trusted persons in on your medical condition, lest there may evolve hurtful and damaging rumors and gossip that are out of your control. The ability to control your own narrative is perhaps the best reason for disclosing your condition to your employer and/ or trusted coworkers so that they may continue to have a realistic view of you based on information that comes straight from you. But, of course, there is no obligation to disclose any medical-related information.

KNOW YOUR RIGHTS (ADA AND FMLA)

You have unique rights regarding employment conferred by having a medical diagnosis like PD. In thinking about your employment, you should consider whether your work position is protected by the Americans with Disabilities Act (ADA). In companies with 15 or more employees, the ADA requires that an employer make reasonable workplace accommodations for someone with a disability rather than terminating their employment. The details of ADA policies are best reviewed with a human resources department; if your company doesn't have one, it's worth speaking to an employment attorney so you are well informed of your rights. Your perspective on the matter should be that discrimination based on a PD diagnosis is not only unfair, it might very well be illegal. There may also be a challenge (albeit a worthwhile one) in changing your employer's well-meaning but incorrect perceptions about PD.

If PD causes you to sometimes require breaks from regular employment, an employer knowledgeable about PD should create accommodations without negotiation. However, it's important to be aware of another work-related federal policy that protects your ability to take time off for legitimate needs, as certified by your physician. This policy is called the Family and Medical Leave Act (FMLA). As its name implies, FMLA establishes guidelines and allowances for being away from work even if "sick leave" has been exhausted or doesn't apply to the particular reasons why you might need time away. Become familiar with the details of this program even if you don't think it is necessary now, as it may be needed down the road.

HEALTH INSURANCE

Health insurance needs for the PD patient are similar to those for others with a comparable health profile. Perhaps the highest priority for planning coverage needs is the cost of outpatient maintenance medications. For those with basic Medicare plans, supplementary coverage for Part D (outpatient medications) can be a valuable investment, since some of the medications used for symptomatic control are brand-name (as opposed to generic) products. For such formulations, the co-pay can be quite high.

DISABILITY AND RETIREMENT

For some persons with PD, consideration and recognition of medical disability may become necessary. The pace of PD progression is generally slow enough that a mild case won't approach a high level of outward symptomatology for several years, if ever. However, eventually some patients may lose sufficient ability to continue with employment. A decision to proceed with a disability application can be the decision of either an employer or a patient; however, the Social Security process acts independently to determine whether the employee applicant meets adequate criteria for full disability and benefits. Disability in the context of PD is sometimes a highly individualized, challenging concept. Sometimes the inability to safely operate a motor vehicle is the key factor for a disability determination. Other factors include impaired balance leading to repeated falls in the work environment, speech impairment in a position requiring verbal communication, or difficulties with dexterity-demanding tasks such as typing and writing. From these examples, it's clear that the process of disability determination is quite specific to the type of employment and whether appropriate accommodations can be made. Employers may be interested in facilitating retirement with medical disability for workers who desire this outcome; however, it is important for the employee to obtain sound advice as to whether short- and long-term disability insurance provided by the employer will be in agreement with human resources policies and whether an assessment by the Social Security review will ultimately lead to the same conclusion. In many communities, legal advice is available from attorneys who are quite familiar with PD in the context of workplace laws, and it is recommended to seek such input in order to be as informed as possible about your rights as an employee.

Social Security Disability Insurance (SSDI) and Supplemental Security Income (SSI) are federally supported benefit programs from the Social Security Administration. These benefit programs are available for persons with PD on the basis of meeting age or disability requirements (or both); each program has specific criteria and limitations. They are part of the social safety net but shouldn't be viewed as taking unfair advantage. SSI is directed at providing financial assistance to adults aged 65 years and older and to persons with disability regardless of age if lacking sufficient income or other resources. Some states have additional supplementation of funds. SSDI offers another means of support for persons who meet certain levels of disability and have a qualifying work history. The credit for prior work can either be their own efforts or from either a spouse or parent.

In most states, a recipient of SSI will also qualify for Medicaid support. Furthermore, if SSDI has been approved, a disabled person with SSDI automatically qualifies for Medicare following

24 months of disability payments. Other rules apply for different disability conditions.

How disability is determined for someone with PD is not always easy to comprehend. Obviously, different occupations interact with disability differently. Short-term or partial disability does not qualify as a situation of eligibility for either SSI or SSDI. The laws and policies governing disability determination may seem arbitrary in some instances. The ability to perform work and the permanency of disability need to be ascertained by review of medical records in support of an application, and an in-person medical evaluation is often needed. The process of application review and decision-making can take, on average, three to five months from the date of application. The appeal process is often needed to reverse an initial determination that a person with PD doesn't qualify. There is also a process to obtain expedited review of disability through the SSI and SSDI Compassionate Allowances program.

For those PD persons who are working, employers may have different views on retaining or retiring workers. Sometimes an employer will show great sympathy to an employee and choose to increase disability benefits or offer full disability benefits (as opposed to retirement benefits). Sometimes not. As you consider what might be your best choices, consultation with an employment attorney might provide useful guidance on the best strategy based on your employment circumstances.

Sexuality and Intimacy

We know now that there are multiple changes, both physical and mental, that can occur in someone with PD. The motor-specific symptoms of PD (and even its nonmotor manifestations) sometimes affect sexuality. For some, there is also a decline in sexual intimacy for many reasons, and sometimes as a consequence of changes in self-image.

At any time during the progression of PD, there can be a change in sexual health, which in turn can affect intimate relationships in several ways. In this section, you'll explore some of the challenges Parkinson's patients may face in staying intimate with their partners and learn about possible treatment options.

MALE SEXUAL HEALTH

For men and women alike, the diagnosis of PD may change the nature of an intimate relationship as well as the physiology of sex between partners. In one dimension, it might be the mechanics, such as difficulties in positioning the body in bed, for example. For males at all ages, erectile dysfunction (ED) leading to impotence is known to be more prevalent in PD patients. This is usually not due to medications typically used to treat PD, though some medications do have side effects leading to ED. Not uncommonly, ED precedes the onset of PD, and it has been reported to be a major risk factor for acquiring PD. PD may also contribute to decreased sexual functioning because it's associated with lower circulating concentrations of the male sex hormone testosterone. This deficiency can contribute to decreased sexual performance and libido. Libido, which refers to a person's interest and drive for engaging in sexual behavior, is known to be reduced in PD to a greater extent than in age-matched men without PD. For this reason, a medical evaluation for problems in male sexual health takes all of these factors into account. Decreased libido and ED are linked to other causes as well, including depression, advanced age, and various neurological conditions, such as peripheral neuropathy and peripheral vascular disease. For most men over the age of 50, intermittent or consistent ED is a relatively common problem. A urological assessment can evaluate the causes of and possible treatments for ED, which include medications that can temporarily and effectively counteract ED and, if needed, supplement testosterone.

Of course, not all male sexual problems that occur in PD patients are explained by the causes just described. Having PD can also affect intimacy by altering self-image, which, in turn, can lessen a PD patient's confidence in an intimate relationship with his partner. The physical signs of PD can contribute to a weakened image of vigor or personal strength. Particularly if a PD patient has progressed to a state of physical dependency on a caregiver, the consequences might include diminished self-worth. Discussions about sharing feelings and working out ways for returning to a confident and satisfying physical relationship are important and can be had with primary care physicians, psychiatrists, psychologists, marriage counselors, and social workers. Be sure to seek a therapist with adequate credentials to serve as a source of credible and trustworthy advice and support.

FEMALE SEXUAL HEALTH

For women with PD, many of the same issues as discussed in the previous section apply. Sometimes libido also declines in women with PD. Often, the onset of PD coincides with menopause, which itself can be a major upset to a secure self-image in a sexual relationship. Of course, romantic love is not all about intercourse or physical attractiveness, and those in long-term relationships generally enjoy strong foundations that allow them to take advantage of resources that can facilitate coping with the physical and sexual discomforts and disabilities of PD.

Just like mobility and dexterity, sexual intimacy can undergo a change after the diagnosis of PD. This change can arise even in the absence of any physical disabilities; it can be linked to altered self-image or a loss of confidence that PD can impose. Some patients have confided in me that PD makes them feel less attractive or "ancient" at an age when they are not old. The one advantage of being a woman with PD is that ED will not be an additional problem. However, as for men, PD can alter the mechanics of sexual performance in women. For some people, changing positions in bed can be difficult. A resting tremor can seem monumental when it comes to sexual excitement. Fortunately, loving couples can often find a way around these difficulties. Despite PD, a sexual relationship can prosper as long as both partners possess a realistic understanding of what it is like to live with PD. This calls for a certain amount of preparatory conversation on the topic, and perhaps some research and consultation with a physician. Those who have studied sexuality in PD (and there is much written about this topic) recognize that major problems expressed by PD patients regarding sex and intimacy are often the same ones expressed by others without PD.

As we've seen, PD affects both men and women in equal measure when it comes to problems with sexual and physical intimacy. Sexual dysfunction, lack of sexual arousal, and a decrease in libido can be common problems, especially in a population that is getting older. However, honest and open conversations, both with your partner and with your health care provider, in addition to realistic understandings of what it means to live with PD, can help PD patients and their partners remain intimately connected in the midst of so much change.

Preserving Your Independence

A few years ago, while I was speaking to a local PD support group and wishing to perk up the audience, I decided to take a vote about renaming PD. The term "disease," however medically appropriate, doesn't sit well with many people who regard themselves, quite rightly, as perfectly healthy despite the label of PD. With this in mind, I took a vote and allowed the majority to rule with their decision that the term "disease" was abolished, at least for that evening. There was a sincere feeling in the room that night that using the term "disease" was too gloomy, too pessimistic for a condition that everyone in the support group was attempting to master in their own ways, and largely succeeding. In fact, this might be the proper perspective, to keep the terminology simple and just call it "Parkinson's." "Take the Parkinson's challenge" is the way that one of my patients described it; whether this means pursuing an aggressive exercise program that satisfies the urge to maintain vitality, or just the intent to become a better communicator with friends and family, a positive personal philosophy can open doors to significantly better living with PD. Of course, being lucky enough to have a mild and nonprogressive form of PD can be a very useful ally in maintaining a positive attitude. An important fact I leave many patients with is that the odds are quite strong for a good outcome. Especially if one's symptoms are asymmetrical or one-sided and resting tremor is a feature, the progression of PD can often be quite slow and extremely responsive to medication. How does one know whether this promising outcome is likely? I have observed that three years after onset of symptoms is a milestone at which patients can predict the outcome of their PD. If, three years after the onset of symptoms, there has been little to no progression of the condition, a milder overall outcome is usually evident at five years and beyond. Of course, this is no guarantee of freedom from worsening symptoms or disability, but realistic optimism is warranted, given the odds in favor of a relatively benign outcome. Take a look at Michael J. Fox's books on his experience living with PD, such as *Lucky Man* and *A Funny Thing Happened on the Way to the Future: Twists and Turns and Lessons Learned*. In these books you can gain a candid and insightful view of the pathway to acceptance and even a sense of liberation about what PD can be despite all of its inconveniences and discomforts.

Who are your peers with PD? In addition to Michael J. Fox, several celebrities have been afflicted—Muhammad Ali, the singer Linda Ronstadt, Pope John Paul II, and Charles Schulz (creator of the *Peanuts* comic strip)—along with some of the nicest people I know. I have sensed that the shared experience of living with the outward manifestations of PD, particularly the tremor and voice impairments, if present, creates a sort of de facto kinship among affected persons, especially in settings such as support group meetings, where these features are well understood. The sense of willingness to help fellow sufferers is never more apparent than in the well-attended PD walks regularly held by local and national PD organizations in an effort to raise research funds, or just to get out the word about resources and support for those living with this disorder. Hundreds of people attend these walks in recognition and celebration of someone's struggle or successful coping with PD. At my community's annual PD walk, the competition among participating teams for who can raise the most money can be fierce!

In the context of PD, maintaining your independence and a satisfying lifestyle may require a reorientation of your personal philosophy. With PD, you become subject to being stereotyped by others—and possibly by yourself, especially if you start to think of yourself as just a "PD patient" rather than a person who happens to have the diagnosis of PD and who nonetheless is making the most of life despite it. Improving your identity may require the bolstering of your identity as a fighter, an activist, or an improved communicator to those around you so that sympathy isn't your mode of interaction with others. Some patients have been successful with a certain amount of denial about their experience with PD. As long as you don't approach it with total denial, this can work, too. Your personal philosophy can be guided by some elements of what PD isn't: a fatal disorder or a disease that robs you of enjoyment in reading a good book, playing with grandchildren, the taste of your favorite ice cream, or the faith you have in a higher power or in your fellow humans. It's not uncommon in conversations with my patients to learn that they have even developed a certain pride in the manner of their coping with PD. Those patients who engage in support group activities (sometimes as leaders) or in Rock Steady Boxing classes, for example, have often told me that these activities for PD patients bring out a satisfying sense of community.

Preserving your independence starts with a sense of self-worth—PD doesn't take away any of that. Persons with PD often express worries that, someday, they might be a burden to their spouse or their children. That may be so, but severe arthritis, heart problems, or any number of other health setbacks will also interfere with independence, and these can happen to any aging person, regardless of PD. The path forward to maintaining a positive attitude is to recognize that most persons with PD do not have significant disabilities at five years postdiagnosis or beyond. These are the fortunate facts, and everyone should become an optimist in the face of the possibility of a less than ideal outcome with PD. Even persons needing some assistance (or patience) from others can still remain largely independent. In the modern era, fewer and fewer people are hiding from family, friends, coworkers, and society in general because of this disorder. If this is not the case for you, then liberating yourself from these concerns should become your goal. Find others who will work with you to make this happen, and surround yourself with them.

CONCLUSION

The introduction of this book included a statement about how I view the challenge of PD: to make the most of currently available treatment options and to develop a better understanding of PD so that affected persons will have a better quality of life. A cure would be nice to have available, as well as improved versions of symptomatic therapies. I hope that I have convinced you, the reader, that these unmet needs are heading toward a solution through research going on worldwide and leading to frequent new developments. Believe me, your life ahead with PD has good odds of success. And for this reason, the world around you doesn't want you to hide from it.

The world around you has an image of PD that might not be as sophisticated as yours if you have studied it. The language we use in talking about human illness has a significant impact on how it is perceived. Both for the patient and for those around them, having a medical diagnosis with the term "disease" is stigmatizing and erodes self-confidence. I sometimes encourage people with PD to dissect this word to gain some insight into why it can strike fear into your everyday life. "Disease" might be one way to analyze why it's such an image problem. Life might be perceived as "easy" if you don't have PD (not so, of course!). But can your life ever return to an "easy" state of feeling healthy? This is one of the challenges ahead for you—with PD, you can be perfectly healthy. You can also take measures to make yourself even healthier. Take a look at what gaps there might be in your personal preventive health management. Are you getting flu shots annually? Are colonoscopies carried out on a recommended schedule for your age and familial risk pattern? Are women getting regular breast exams and Pap smears, and men getting appropriate prostate examinations? Are tests of your blood pressure and lipid profile showing that you are in the normal range? Are you getting regular dermatology examinations? Your compliance with these and other health assessments is important to consider if you wish to be proactive in avoiding medical problems. Checking the boxes on your personal health monitoring might, I hope, be a source of "easing" your worries about the health impact that PD imposes on you.

One of the many insights I have learned from PD patients is that resilience can come from many sources. It can come from others living with PD, which is why I am always in favor of seeking out a PD support group. It can also come from learning even more about PD than this book has provided. Sometimes good social support and the good fortune of having relatively mild PD make it easier to live a full and productive life despite the intrusion of PD. I hope you, the reader, are just that person.

RESOURCES

Suggested Reading

Ahlskog, J. Eric. *The New Parkinson's Disease Treatment Book: Partnering with Your Doctor to Get the Most from Your Medications.* 2nd ed. New York: Oxford University Press, 2015.

An authoritative, updated account by a senior Mayo Clinic PD specialist. Not overly technical, but more information than many people might feel they need.

Dorros, Sidney. *Parkinson's: A Patient's View.* Cabin John, MD: Seven Locks Press, 1981. (Out of print, but widely available through secondhand book sources in its hardcover or paperback editions.)

One of the earliest first-person accounts of experiencing and coping with PD. Sid Dorros developed PD at age 40, anticipating it because both his parents were also affected. He brought a rare insight to understanding the process of accepting and mastering PD with practical suggestions and a sense of humor. Well worth seeking out.

Fox, Michael J. *A Funny Thing Happened on the Way to the Future: Twists and Turns and Lessons Learned.* New York: Hyperion Books, 2010.

The actor, activist for Parkinson's disease, and founder of the most successful foundation for fostering PD research tells his life story of acquiring this illness at age 30. An inspiring tale of how one person with PD has helped so many others. He also published a second book, Lucky Man, *which I also recommend.*

Marie, Lianna. *Everything You Need to Know about Parkinson's Disease: The Complete Guide for People with Parkinson's and Their Caregivers*. rev. ed. CreateSpace, 2015.

By the daughter of a PD patient, this volume lives up to its title and provides a diverse range of practical tips and solid information. Other publications by the author can be found at www.allaboutparkinsons.com.

Palfreman, Jon. *Brain Storms: The Race to Unlock the Mysteries of Parkinson's Disease*. New York: Scientific American / Farrar, Straus and Giroux, 2015.

The author is a seasoned journalist, educator, and television producer. He takes an in-depth look at the latest research developments with the insight of a scientist and as a person affected with PD. Take a look at his op-ed about his personal PD experience, entitled "The Bright Side of Parkinson's" (New York Times, February 21, 2015), and other writings.

Peterman Schwarz, Shelley. *Parkinson's Disease: 300 Tips for Making Life Easier*. 2nd ed. New York: Demos Medical Publishing, 2006.

An accomplished writer on disability and human nature takes on PD. The 300 tips cover a wide range of topics pertaining to safety, convenience, and other everyday matters.

Pickut, Barbara, Sven Vanneste, Mark A. Hirsch, Wim Van Hecke, Eric Kerckhofs, Peter Mariën, Paul M. Parizel, David Crosiers, and Patrick Cras. "Mindfulness Training among Individuals with Parkinson's Disease: Neurobehavioral Effects." *Parkinson's Disease* (2015): 816404. doi.org/10.1155/2015/816404.

As discussed in chapter 5 (page 87), this is an investigation of the impact of mindfulness on PD symptoms.

Websites with Information about Parkinson's Disease

American Parkinson Disease Association (Staten Island, NY; APDAParkinson.org)

ClinicalTrials.gov (repository of information about all ongoing PD clinical research in the United States and internationally)

Cure Parkinson's Trust (London, UK; CureParkinsons.org.uk)

Davis Phinney Foundation (DavisPhinneyFoundation.org)

LSVT Global: an organization that offers evidence-based speech, physical, and occupational therapies for people with Parkinson's and other conditions (LSVTGlobal.com)

Michael J. Fox Foundation for Parkinson's Research (New York, NY; MichaelJFox.org)

Parkinson Canada (Toronto, ON; Parkinson.ca)

Parkinson's Foundation (Miami, FL; Parkinson.org)

Parkinson's UK (London, UK; Parkinsons.org.uk)

World Health Organization: Depression fact sheet (WHO.int/news-room/fact-sheets/detail/depression)

World Parkinson Congress (WorldPDCongress.org)

INDEX

Progressive supranuclear palsy
(PSP), 13–14
Psychologists, 47–48

R
Registered dietitians (RDs), 48–49
Relationships, 74–76. *See also*
Intimacy
Retirement, 95–97
Ronstadt, Linda, 102

S
Schulz, Charles, 102
Self-compassion, 86–87
Sexual health
female, 99–101
male, 98–99
"Sick role," 74
Sinemet, 53
Sleep, 26
Smell, sense of, 27–28, 29
Social Security Disability
Insurance (SSDI), 96–97
Social workers, 50–51

Speech, 24
Speech therapists, 46–47
Striatum, 6, 28, 51
Supplemental Security Income
(SSI), 96–97
Support groups, 80–81, 84
Support teams, 67–70
Surgical interventions, 58–64
Symptoms, 21–23
motor, 23–25, 27
nonmotor, 27–28

T
Thalamotomy, 60–62
Tools for daily activities, 82–83
Tremors, 7, 25, 67–68, 93

U
Uric acid, 31

W
Wilson's disease, 14
Workplace, 90–91, 93–97

ABOUT THE AUTHOR

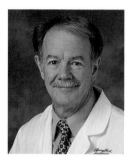 **Peter LeWitt, MD,** is a board-certified neurologist and has directed the Parkinson's Disease and Movement Disorders Center at Henry Ford Hospital in West Bloomfield, Michigan, since 2007. In 1990, he was appointed professor of neurology at Wayne State University's School of Medicine, where he holds an endowed chair in PD research. In addition to extensive experience in conducting clinical trials for PD and other neurological disorders, his research interests have included animal models and biomarkers of neurological disease, pharmacokinetic analysis of neurological drugs, and gene therapy. He is the author of more than 300 publications in basic and clinical neuroscience, most of them related to PD.